Decision–Making for the Periodontal Team

Quintessentials of Dental Practice – 11
Periodontology - 2

Decision-Making
for the Periodontal Team

By
Suzanne Noble
Margaret Kellett
Iain Chapple

Editor-in-Chief: Nairn H F Wilson
Editor Periodontology: Iain LC Chapple

Quintessence Publishing Co. Ltd.

London, Berlin, Chicago, Copenhagen, Paris, Milan, Barcelona,
Istanbul, São Paulo, Tokyo, New Dehli, Moscow, Prague, Warsaw

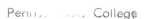
British Library Cataloguing in Publication Data

Noble, Suzanne
  Decision making for the periodontal team. - (Quintessentials of dental practice ;
11. Periodontology ; 2)
  1. Periodontics 2.Dental teams – decision making
  I. Title II. Kellett, Margaret III. Chapple, Iain L. (Iain Leslie)
  617.6′32

ISBN 1850970637

ISBN 1-85097-063-7

*Dedicated to our families
and our patients*

Foreword

Decision-making for the Periodontal Team - Volume 11 and the second periodontology book in the Quintessentials of Dental Practice Series, is a timely
publication. The dental team is about to come of age with GDC registration of the professions complementary to dentistry, and now is the time to
stand back and critically review the quality of the team approach to patient
care in your practice. Where better to start than periodontology?

Dental hygienists, not to forget all the other members of the dental team,
can substantially influence the oral health of your patients and, in turn, their
satisfaction with the service provided by your practice. The extent to which
you, as team leader, and your staff plan the care of patients together, and
work and communicate as a team, will determine the extent to which your
patients' oral health will benefit from team dentistry. Working together in
an appropriate, well-managed practice environment is of fundamental
importance to meeting patients' needs and ever-increasing expectations.
This together with sound, evidence-based decisions in relation to treatment
can turn a good practice into a highly successful practice in which patients
have confidence.

Are you confident in deciding what forms of periodontal care are best for
your patients? When do you refer a patient with periodontal problems to a
specialist periodontologist? How do other forms of treatment - for example,
advanced restorative care, orthodontics and implant therapy - impact on
periodontal health and relevant treatment regimes? Above all else, it is your
responsibility to avoid the situation where the teeth and restorations have
been made good for years to come, but the periodontium is diseased, dete-
riorating and running the risk of entering terminal decline.

If this brief foreword has touched on issues that have made you stop and
think, or you know need to be addressed in your practice, this compact fact-
and guideline-filled book will be a very sound investment.

Nairn Wilson
Editor-in-Chief

Preface

In order for the dental profession to deliver high quality care for patients, an appropriately skilled team is required. Within recent years the General Dental Council specialist lists have been established and the number of registered dental hygienists has increased. Many general dental practitioners are now in a position to select the most appropriate skilled personnel for specific phases of patient management.

For the care plan to be successful, the patient must be educated about the role each member of the team will take in his or her management. It is the general dental practitioner's responsibility to co-ordinate the team and take overall responsibility as the team leader. He or she also has a legal responsibility for procedures delegated to team members who are not registered dentists. It is a professional requirement of each dentist to delegate to professionals complementary to dentistry (PCDs) only those tasks which the person concerned is trained and competent to undertake. Competence implies not only the legal qualification to perform a skilled procedure but the ability to perform that skill to a recognised professional standard without supervision. Members of the team who have not had the opportunity to practise a procedure regularly will become "de-skilled". General dental practitioners therefore need to be mindful of competence before delegating tasks and to support the continual professional development (CPD) of their team.

The overall treatment plan should not only encompass the management of the periodontal disease, but the integration of other specialities in order to achieve a stable, functional, aesthetic masticatory unit, which the patient can maintain. This book will guide the general dental practitioner through the decision-making process for the periodontal team.

This book can be read separately from the other four in the periodontal series. However, reference will be made to the other books, as the series is designed to develop certain aspects and concepts and to reinforce these throughout the process.

Acknowledgements

The authors are grateful for the help of the following people. In Birmingham, Marina Tipton helped with the photography and Helena Smith with the manuscript. Thanks to Stewart Hawkins for proof-reading Chapter 2 and to Pharmacia Limited for guidance on the Nicorette® products and for providing Fig 5-14. Thanks to Dr Adrian Shorthall for use of Fig 9-7. In Leeds, thanks to Mr PA Cook, Mr JK Williams and Mr L Boyle for loan of clinical slides, to Ian Smith for scanning electron microscopy and to John Walker for photographic assistance.

Contents

The Periodontal Team

Aim

This chapter aims to provide the general dental practitioner (GDP) with an insight into the development and role of professionals complementary to dentistry within the context of the management of periodontal diseases.

Outcome

As a result of reading this chapter the practitioner should have an under-standing of how the periodontal team has evolved and the legally permitted duties of dental hygienists and dental therapists.

Introduction

It is in the primary care setting that the vast majority of periodontal disease is diagnosed and managed. The *team* involved in patient care may be small, involving only the dentist, dental hygienist and dental nurse. Conversely, the team may work together in a large polyclinic where periodontal care is one of many specialist dental services offered. In such situations the periodontal specialist will be available for the diagnosis and management of the more complex cases.

In its broadest sense, the dental team reaches beyond the high street surgery to include the secondary care services in hospital periodontal departments where the consultant in restorative dentistry and his or her team will offer advice and, where appropriate, treatment of referred cases.

In order to obtain the most appropriate care for an individual patient the GDP will refer the patient to other team members to utilise their skills, knowledge and experience to achieve the desired treatment outcomes. Rather than this referral process being considered as a hierarchical model, it is suggested that it be considered in a circular form with the GDP at the centre. It is the GDP with whom the patient is registered and it is the GDP to whom the patient returns for continuing care (Fig 1-1). The role of the GDP is an *infinite* one! The other team members have important skills to offer, but

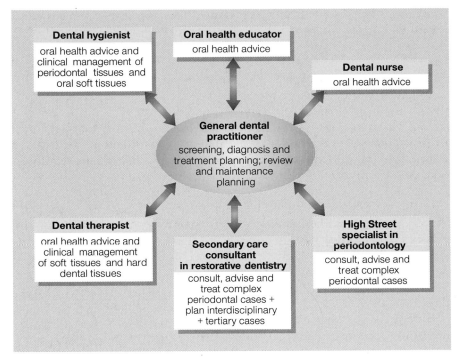

Fig 1-1 Members of the periodontal team.

their roles are *finite* ones, clearly defined by the practitioner's referral request or treatment plan.

By co-ordinating the referral process the practitioner plays the key role in consolidating the treatment and ensuring that the patient is informed of the reasons behind the referral. The role of the practitioner as the team leader is explored further in Chapter 3, but by way of introduction to "working together" this chapter will focus on the evolution of the professionals complementary to dentistry and the skills these team members have to offer.

The Dental Hygienist

Although dental hygienists were first trained in the United States in 1913, there was no formal training in the UK until 1943, in the Royal Air Force. During the next 20–30 years schools of dental hygiene were founded and attached to dental schools, but they trained relatively few hygienists compared to dentists. Enrolment with the General Dental Council (GDC) became mandatory in 1957.

The original concepts of *patient education* and *prevention* of periodontal diseases remain the linchpin of the dental hygienist's role, but the range of permitted duties has expanded in recent years in line with the current concepts of team management for patients with oral diseases. Dually qualified dental hygienists/therapists now receive education to diploma and degree levels in universities alongside undergraduate dental students. This enhances the periodontal team concept within the workplace.

The changing patterns of oral disease and the increasing public awareness and demand for oral health was the driver behind the *Nuffield Inquiry into Education and Training of Personnel Auxiliary to Dentistry* in 1993. This extensive inquiry examined the role of dental auxiliary personnel, and stimulated widespread debate on a number of key issues surrounding the development of the dental team. Following this the GDC set up the Dental Auxiliaries Review Group (DARG), to prepare appropriate recommendations in relation to all classes of dental auxiliary. The committee reported in 1998, setting out proposals on permitted duties, entry requirements and registration. It was also recommended that the team concept for future practice should be promoted through the training of dentists and dental auxiliaries in close association with each other.

Subsequently, in 1999, the GDC announced a new era for professionals complementary to dentistry. The council supported statutory registration of all members of the dental team and the widening of clinical roles after appropriate education and training. Although the term *dental hygienist* remained protected, as it was a role with which the general public was familiar, the dental hygienist became incorporated into a wider group subsequently named Professionals Complementary to Dentistry (PCD). The GDC emphasised that entry to the register would be on the basis of appropriate education and that each PCD should practise only under the delegated authority of a registered dentist.

It was the expressed intention of the GDC that all PCDs should continue to work within the dental team within which the dentist would remain responsible for diagnosis, treatment planning and the quality control of the treatment provided (Fig 1-2).

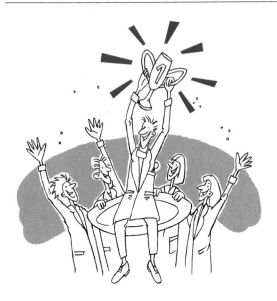

Fig 1-2 The team and team leader.

Legally Permitted Duties

Until such time as the GDC is able to register all PCDs, dental hygienists and dental therapists may practise dentistry to the extent of the Dentists Act 1984 and the 1986 Dental Auxiliaries Regulations, with amendments in 1991 and 2002. It is an offence to practise outside these limits.

They are permitted to work "under the direction of a registered dentist". This implies that the dentist has examined the patient and indicated in writing the course of treatment to be provided. The dentist need not necessarily be present on the premises at the time the hygienist or therapist is carrying out the treatment. This legislation formed part of the 1991 amendment to permit hygienists to carry out domiciliary visits.

The supervisory role of the dentist varies in differing clinical situations and it is the dentist's responsibility to be aware of these parameters. In the case of treatment of a patient under conscious sedation by a hygienist or therapist, the dentist must be in the surgery with the patient throughout treatment. Whilst inferior dental nerve blocks are being administered the dentist must be on the premises but not necessarily in the room. With the introduction of expanded duties from 2002, many practitioners will be involved in workplace post-qualification training for additional skills for hygienists and therapists, and the recommendations are for close personal supervision of a designated number of procedures.

Dental hygienists are permitted to carry out the following kinds of dental work:
- Cleaning and polishing teeth.
- Scaling teeth (i.e. the removal of deposits, accretions and stains from those parts of the surfaces of the teeth which are exposed or which are directly beneath the free margins of the gums, including the application of appropriate medicaments).
- The application to the teeth of such prophylactic materials as the GDC may from time to time determine.
- Giving advice within the meaning of section 37(1) of the Dentists Act 1984 such as may be necessary for the proper performance of the dental work prescribed.
- The taking of dental radiographs.
- The administration of local infiltration and inferior dental nerve block analgesia for the purpose of scaling or root debridement.
- The taking of impressions for diagnostic purposes.
- The emergency placement of temporary dressings and replacement of crowns with temporary cement.
- The treatment of patients under conscious sedation.

Depending upon the date of primary qualification, there may be additional skills obtained and certified by course attendance and workplace supervision. In clinical practice the dental hygienist's skills include:
- The removal of supra- and subgingival calculus.
- Closed root surface debridement (RSD).
- Appropriate oral hygiene advice.
- The application of local delivery antimicrobial agents as an adjunct in periodontal therapy (under the Medicines Act 1968 the dentist must prescribe the drug to be used).
- Management of dentinal hypersensitivity with appropriate medicaments.
- Prevention of dental caries by the application of topical fluoride.
- Fissure sealing (the use of filled resins in minimally prepared cavities is not permitted).
- Polishing dental restorations.

Dental therapists may carry out all the duties listed for dental hygienists with the addition of:
- Extraction of deciduous teeth.

- Simple fillings.
- Pulp therapy to deciduous teeth.
- The placement of prefabricated crowns on deciduous teeth.

Permitted Duties of Dental Hygienists and Dental Therapists since the 1986 Dental Auxiliaries Regulations

Local anaesthesia

Local infiltration analgesia
Dental hygienists who hold the Diploma in Dental Hygiene awarded after 1992, or dental therapists who hold the Diploma in Dental Therapy (formerly the Certificate of Proficiency) may carry out scaling under local infiltration analgesia. This competency was included in the hygienists' core curriculum from 1992 onwards. Therefore hygienists qualifying after that date will not hold separate certification.

Dental hygienists who qualified before 1992 must to be able to demonstrate competency by presentation of a certificate proving post-qualification training in local infiltration analgesia. Following legislation passed on 1 July 2002, the dentist does not have to be on the premises whilst the dental hygienist is administering local infiltration analgesia. *Under these circumstances a third person with current training in cardiopulmonary resuscitation must be on the premises.*

Inferior nerve block regional analgesia
Following the July 2002 amendments to the regulations, dental hygienists and therapists are permitted to carry out their statutory duties under the administration of an inferior dental block that they have personally administered. The recommendations are that the training period must include 10 closely supervised procedures in the workplace before certification by the awarding authority is issued. *Following this, a registered dentist must be on the premises whenever an inferior dental block is administered by a dental hygienist or therapist.*

Dental radiography

Dental hygienists and dental therapists may take dental radiographs provided they have received training according to the Ionising Radiation Medical Exposure Regulations IR(ME)R 2000.

Since July 1992 dental radiography has been included in the core curriculum for dental hygienists. Those persons who qualified prior to this date must undergo the recognised training and have evidence of certification to be legally permitted to take radiographs. The courses of training are similar to those undertaken by dental nurses.

The emergency placement of temporary dressings and replacement of crowns with temporary cement
Providing the dental hygienist or dental therapist has undergone appropriate training (according to the regulations of 1999 and 2002) they may place a temporary filling material or replace a crown with temporary cement provided that the filling or crown was dislodged whilst they were treating the patient. The regulations state that both the patient and the dentist must be informed of the event and the patient must be advised to see the dentist as soon as possible.

Impression taking
Similar to the above, according to the 2002 regulations, providing that the dental hygienist or dental therapist has undergone appropriate training they may take impressions for study models. The recommendations are that following theoretical training five sets of impressions must be undertaken with the supervision of the dentist, or an appropriately trained and certified dental hygienist or therapist, in the workplace before certification will be issued by the awarding authority.

Treatment of patients under conscious sedation
Dental hygienists and therapists may treat patients according to their remit under conscious sedation provided they have undergone appropriate training in a recognised educational establishment, and *always* with the dentist in the surgery at the time the procedure is being carried out.

Sectors of Dentistry

Dental hygienists have always been able to work in all sectors of dentistry, but dental therapists were restricted to practise in the Public Health Services and the Personal Dental Service pilot schemes. Since the revised regulations of July 2002 dental therapists may work in all sectors of dentistry.

As stated previously, it is illegal for dental hygienists and therapists to practise dentistry other than is permitted by the Dentists Act 1984 and the 1986 Dental Auxiliary regulations and amendments. In this regard, it is unlawful for the dentist to prescribe treatment which does not fall within the permitted duties, neither is it appropriate that these persons are directed to work in an unreasonable manner. Both parties may be liable to a charge of misconduct if this situation arises.

The prescription from the dentist to the hygienist or therapist must be understood by all concerned, without risk of ambiguity. It is a medicolegal requirement that prescriptions are signed and dated by the prescriber and retained with the case notes. The patient must be examined by a dentist every 12 months although interim treatments between these examinations are permissible.

Ethical Guidance/Maintaining Standards

In terms of what the public, patients and the professions expect, the GDC directs hygienists and therapists towards their ethical guidance – maintenance of standards. Failure to follow this guidance may lead to a charge of misconduct (i.e. any behaviour which adversely reflects on the professions, such as dishonesty, indecency, violence, alcohol or drug abuse (Fig 1-3); giving untrue, misleading or unethical statements, particularly when interacting with the media; and abuse of the relationship between the patient and clinician, particularly with regard to trust and maintaining confidentiality).

Dental hygienists and dental therapists must obtain informed consent for any treatment they undertake, update the patient's medical history and inform

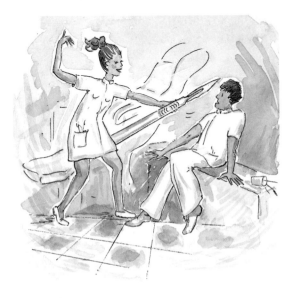

Fig 1-3 Adverse behaviour.

the dentist of any changes. They must provide a high standard of care by always acting in the best interests of the patient and keep full and up-to-date records of all treatment.

It is the responsibility of the prescribing dentist as well as the hygienist or therapist to ensure that a third party is present on the premises whenever treatment is undertaken – this includes domiciliary visits.

The dental hygienist and therapist must be fully aware of the practice protocols on infection control. Any breach of national guidelines is likely to lead to a charge of misconduct both for the operator and the practice owner.

It is imperative that dental hygienists and dental therapists are fully prepared to deal with a medical emergency. It is their responsibility to ensure training is regularly updated and certified. It is the dentist's responsibility to provide the mandatory resuscitation equipment and to ensure all the team members practise resuscitation routines in a simulated emergency situation.

In the future, the statutory list of permitted duties is likely to be replaced by regulation through curricula, ethical guidance and professional responsibility to practise dentistry within the limits of competence. This concept develops a framework of responsibility with flexibility. The dentist has overall responsibility for the patient's oral care plan, while delegating aspects of treatment to a suitability trained and qualified PCD. The PCD would be professionally accountable for these specific, delegated requirements.

Key Points of Clinical Relevance

- Patients expect high standards of treatment.
- The treatment should be delivered by an appropriately skilled dental team.
- The team must be led and co-ordinated by the dentist.
- All members have an obligation to be committed to self-audit and continuing professional and personal development.
- The dental surgeon must designate the work to be undertaken by means of a written prescription.

References

General Dental Council Dental Auxiliaries Review Group. London: General Dental Council, 1998.

Nuffield Inquiry into Education and Training of Personnel Auxiliary to Dentistry. London: Nuffield Foundation, 1993.

Further Reading

General Dental Council. Ethical Guidance for Dental Hygienists and Dental Therapists. London: General Dental Council, 2000.

General Dental Council. Professionals Complementary to Dentistry. A Consultation Paper. London: General Dental Council, 1998.

Chapter 2

Medicolegal Aspects of Employing Professionals Complementary to Dentistry

Aim

The aim of this chapter is to guide the practitioner through the recruitment and retention of staff who will form a coherent and effective dental team.

Outcome

As a result of reading this chapter the practitioner should have an awareness of the responsibilities involved in the employment of PCDs.

The Role of the General Dental Council

Several references to the General Dental Council are made throughout the book and it is therefore pertinent to begin this chapter with a brief overview of the role of the GDC:

- Protecting the public by the regulation of dental professionals in the United Kingdom.
- Registering dentists and PCDs.
- Maintaining high standards of personal and professional conduct.
- Ensuring high standards in dental education.
- Requiring dentists to take part in continuing professional development.
- Taking action in the case of concern over a dental professional's fitness to practise.

The Role of the Employer

The practice principal is the employer of staff and consequently has to comply with employment legislation. It is not the role of this book to consider all aspects of employment but to highlight relevant aspects of the employment and management of PCDs in the primary care setting.

Recruitment

The dentist may legally designate almost all non-surgical management of periodontal disease to a dental hygienist or dually qualified dental therapist. The new employee will of course require the provision of a suitably equipped surgery and access to the support of a dental nurse (Chapter 4).

Recruitment is currently difficult due to the limited resource of qualified dental hygienists and therapists. These personnel are trained in relatively small numbers compared to undergraduate dentists and the vast majority are women who, owing to domestic and economic factors, may not be versatile in their geographic location when seeking employment. In a study by Hillam (2000), spanning a 21-year period, of graduates from Liverpool School of Dental Hygiene, only 6% recorded any difficulty finding jobs and 83% reported job satisfaction. The majority work in general dental practice and data suggest they are likely to continue to work in their chosen career, at least as long as female dentists do in theirs.

Bearing these factors in mind, the practitioner must decide whether to advertise locally or nationally. The British Dental Hygienists Association (BDHA) and the British Association of Dental Therapists, (BADT) publish journals in which advertisements may be placed (Fig 2-1). Contacting training schools or word of mouth via friends and colleagues may also be productive. Care must be taken, in the latter situation, not to breach the equal opportunities legislation.

The more information given in the advertisement, the better informed the potential applicant will be, and consequently the employer will not waste time interviewing staff who do not fulfil the required criteria. The majority of dental hygienists work part-time in one or more practices and may not be able to accommodate specific day requirements. Flexibility of days and hours will broaden the potential recruitment base.

Write a job description and a person specification
A written job description and person specification will fulfil two important purposes. The potential applicant will be informed of the details of the post and this will form the basis of the contract of employment later. The person specification allows the employer to reference criteria required against qualifications, experience and personal qualities offered by the applicant. It also provides the evidence for shortlisting for interview.

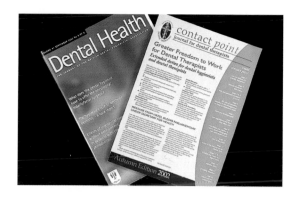

Fig 2-1 Journals of the British Dental Hygienists Association and the British Association of Dental Therapists.

The practice may prefer the completion of a customised application form or request the applicant to submit a current curriculum vitae from which to cross check their qualifications. Issues, which may be explored at interview, are the work experience, in particular any gaps in the employment records, and the applicant's continued professional development record. An applicant who is well prepared would present a portfolio of verification of courses recently attended. The applicant should also indicate two persons who may be contacted for references, one of whom should be the current employer, or in the case of new graduates, an authorised school official.

Arranging the interview

It is courteous to set time aside to interview applicants to allow a full discussion and questions. Whilst a tour of the practice during the working day is very helpful to the applicant, it is not appropriate to conduct the interview during a surgery session. A room should be designated and an interview panel selected. Each member should have decided, in advance, the issues they wish to explore and a chairperson should be appointed to co-ordinate the interview. It is not necessary to ask the applicants the same questions, but it helps if the questions are similar, because this enables objective comparisons to be made and the responses formulated into a numerical score. The questions should not be discriminatory on any grounds, e.g. sex, culture, religion or age. The interview should not be conducted in:

- the surgery whilst working
- the reception area where the patients may overhear
- a setting that is too informal (Fig 2-2).

The following should all be clarified during the interview:

- Terms and conditions of service.

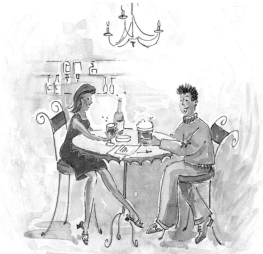

"So, what do you like to do in your spare time?"

Fig 2-2 Not the ideal environment for an interview.

- Equipment provision.
- Nursing support.
- Appointment scheduling.
- Practice protocols.
- Training and development.
- Method of remuneration.

The applicant as well as the employer needs time to reflect, therefore it is normal to inform the applicant when a decision will be made and by what method they will be informed. Be honest. If there are others to interview there is no harm in telling the applicant. The interpretation of references by potential future employers may vary, but if they are not pursued, then the option of obtaining information about the applicant before making a decision is closed.

Offer of employment
This must be in writing, outlining the terms of service and a suggested date for commencement. The employer should request confirmation in writing from the future employee. It is also courteous to inform unsuccessful candidates.

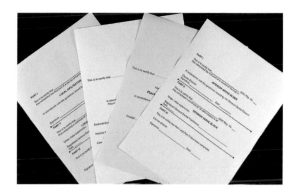

Fig 2-3 Post-qualification certificates.

Document verification

Every employee should have a personal file in which copies of documents are held.

The employer must have sight of the following original documents, of which photocopies are taken for the personal file.

1. The current General Dental Council annual practising certificate (dental hygienists and therapists re-register at the same time as dentists in the UK. PCDs may not practise under a name other than that with which they are registered).
2. Indemnity against claims for professional negligence through verification of current membership of a dental defence organisation (this forms part of the GDC's code of practice for PCDs).
3. Post-qualification certification (expanded duties) The type will depend upon the year of the primary qualification (Fig 2-3). *The GDC does not record these additional qualifications; it is therefore the employer's responsibility to verify the certification.* These may include:
   - local infiltration analgesia
   - radiography
   - insertion of temporary dressings and temporary recementation of crowns
   - inferior dental nerve blocks
   - impression taking
   - conscious sedation.
4. For *all* employees:
   - Evidence of cardiopulmonary resuscitation training within the past 12 months.
   - A record of CPD.

- Evidence of the current HBV antibody titre status (>100 mIU ml^{-1}) and evidence of a booster injection within the past five years.
- Clearance by the Criminal Records Bureau – this is particularly important for staff who will have contact with children and vulnerable adults.

Contract of employment

Generic contracts of employment are available from the BDA, which may be modified according to the practice requirements. This should be agreed and signed by both parties, and a copy given to the employee within two months of commencing work.

Employed verses self-employed status

The law does not define employment or self-employment. This is dependent upon individual cases and important consequences depend upon the label attached to the working relationship by the parties involved. This label may be tested under common law by looking at the contract and tests applied. The standard of the burden of proof is on "a balance of probabilities" (i.e. greater than 50% probability). The Inland Revenue or the Contributions Agency may challenge the working status.

The worker may be an *employee*, i.e. bound by a contract of services, or *self-employed*, i.e. bound by a contract to provide services.

Employee status

An employee is an individual who has entered into or works under a contract of employment (Employment Protection Act 1978). The employer and employee form a contract of service, which carries with it employment rights under employment legislation, especially with regard to dismissal, redundancy payments and maternity rights. It is the employer's responsibility to deduct income tax and National Insurance contributions from the employee at source. Such a contract entitles the employee to social security benefits.

Employed or self-employed?

One of the issues in the debate is the degree of control exercisable by the employer. The greater the degree of employment control exercisable by the employer the more likely it will be that the contract is one of service (see Singh 1995).

Examples of control of the principal dentist over the hygienist/therapist include the premises designated as the place of work, the set hours, hourly, weekly or monthly payment and entitlement to annual leave. The dental hygienist also cannot subcontract which is a recognised practice in self-employment.

The second area for discussion arises around the degree of risk. Hygienists and therapists do not invest in a practice or in the purchase of equipment, nor are they responsible for equipment maintenance. The investment factor favours the employment relationship. The principal appoints and dismisses staff and is responsible for tax deduction. Hygienists and therapists do not, therefore, have control of staff.

The Entrepreneurial Test or Multiple Test asks:
- Is he/she in the business on her/his own?
- Does she/he provide their own equipment?
- Is there any degree of financial responsibility for investment or degree of risk?
- Does he/she undertake any other sort of commissions, business or employment?
- Is there any opportunity to profit from sound management?

This test provides the greatest obstacle to dental hygienists if they are challenged regarding self-employment declaration. For self-employed status to be substantiated the contract between the parties must be clear regarding:
- provision of services for several dentists at different premises
- no regular hours
- selection of own holidays
- providing own equipment
- receiving a percentage of the fees
- able to subcontract to provide a substitute in times of absence.

Employment of persons who have not qualified in the UK
In order for any dental hygienist or therapist to work in the United Kingdom they must be registered with the GDC. Hygienists who have qualified from a country belonging to the European Union (EU) may work in the UK without undertaking any further training, providing they have a good command of the English language and they are on the register.[1] Verification of competence in the English language can be obtained from several sources. One such source is the International English Language Testing System (IELTS). This test encompasses fluency in speaking, listening, reading and writing English.

---

[1] Dental therapists are not trained in any other countries within the European Union.

The professional registration process involves a visit in person to the GDC by the dental hygienist with the original qualification document, birth certificate and marriage certificate if appropriate, and payment of the statutory fee.

Dental hygienists and dental therapists from non-EU countries must undertake a period of additional training before passing the appropriate examination awarded by a university or a Royal College and subsequently applying for registration. The GDC vets the primary qualification and recommends a minimal period of training in a UK school. Dentists who have qualified from non-EU countries are not permitted to work as dental hygienists or dental therapists without undertaking the core training and passing the subsequent diploma examination.

Induction of the New Employee

The principal should designate a member of staff to oversee the induction programme (Box 2-1). The new employee will need time to become familiar with the new environment. Allowing time for administration on the first day will pay dividends in the long term and avoid misunderstandings and errors, which will take longer to rectify (Fig 2-4).

Appraisal

Approximately one month after commencement it is advisable to discuss informally the progress of the new employee. This gives the employee and the employer the opportunity to discuss and clarify issues and to encourage development and participation in the team. Appraisals are subsequently carried out annually, when there is a review of the objectives achieved during the period and a discussion of the development plan for the ensuing 12 months.

Every member of staff should create their own personal file to be kept in their possession. They should also develop a personal development plan, both short term (next 12 months) and longer term (next 3–4 years). The staff should complete the record themselves and copies of all appraisal summaries and CPD certification should be retained on their personal file. The staff member should also have a copy of the appropriate summary, jointly agreed by their employer/manager.

Although CPD is not yet a GDC requirement for PCDs, it is evidence of good practice and will become mandatory in the future.

Box 2-1

Induction Check List
Practice layout
Location of emergency equipment
Protocols
> *health and safety at work and radiation protection*
> *investment in training and development*
> *timing of staff meetings*

Computer systems
Appointment systems
> *record-keeping and information technology training*

Referral policies
Cancellation and failed appointment policies
Operation of equipment
Infection control
Clinical audit
Reporting of sickness and other absences
Risk management protocols, e.g. adverse events log
COSHH (Control of Substances Hazardous to Health)
Practice manuals

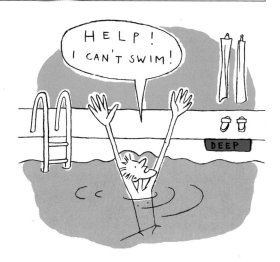

Fig 2-4 Allow time for acclimatisation on the first day.

The guidelines for dentists (250 hours of CPD required over a five-year period with a mix of general and verifiable CPD) will be applied to PCDs. At least 75 of the 250 hours must be spent on undertaking verifiable CPD and the remainder may be general CPD. The GDC's educational criteria for verifiable CPD include:

• concise educational aims and objectives
• clear anticipated outcomes
• quality control – the participant must have an opportunity to comment with a view to improving quality.

Proof of attendance or involvement in verifiable CPD must be available in the form of a certificate or course registration document.

Investment by the practice principal in financially supporting the dental hygienist or dental therapist on courses will reap reward in terms of fulfilled staff. In England, dental hygienists and dental therapists do not receive notification of courses organised by regional postgraduate deaneries, which are circulated only to dentists through the local primary care trusts (PCTs). They are, however, eligible to attend these courses, and as there is no course fee, it is a worthwhile opportunity. The principal can do much to bring to the attention of staff the existence of these courses and attending courses as a team helps develop new practice protocols and teamwork. Dental hygienists have expressed their disappointment in the current underprovision of post-qualification courses. Part of the problem is that they are unable to access the published information on courses for dentists. The majority of courses on periodontology would be suitable for hygienists/therapists to attend. Course organisers are now placing more emphasis on team training, which should encourage attendance. Both the British Dental Hygienists Association (BDHA) and British Association of Dental Therapists (BADT) hold national and regional meetings for their members.

Professional journals
Hygienists and therapists working in general dental practice have limited opportunity to access refereed dental journals. They may join certain specialist societies, and membership would entitle them to journal distribution but the cost may be a deterrant. However, learned societies such as the British Society of Periodontology (BSP) offer hygienists and therapists their services as "associates" of the society at subsidised rates (33%). The BSP also offer reduced subscription rates for associates at national and international meetings and their regional educational programme is available on their website. The electronic journals provide a cheaper option for keeping up to date with the literature.

Useful websites

The following websites have information concerning courses and publications.
- British Society of Periodontology: www.bsperio.org
- British Dental Association: www.bda-dentistry.org.uk
- Royal College of Surgeons of England: www.rcseng.ac.uk
- Royal College of Surgeons of Edinburgh: www.rcsed.ac.uk
- Royal College of Surgeons of Glasgow: www.rcpsglasg.ac.uk

Clinical audit

The appraisal meeting is an opportunity to discuss a potential audit project on which the dental hygienist or therapist may take the lead. This can then be reported to the team at a practice meeting and recommended changes to existing protocols agreed.

Peer review between hygienists and therapists in practices at different locations is a further focus point for clinical audit.

Key Points of Clinical Relevance

It is the principal dentist's responsibility
- To comply with employment legislation and the GCD's guidelines.
- To keep up-to-date records of all staff.
- To obtain a copy of the annual practising certificate of all persons on the PCD register in January of each year.
- To obtain annual verification of professional indemnity insurance.
- To obtain annual verification of cardio pulmonary resuscitation training.
- To verify additional training of PCDs from time to time.
- To encourage all members of the team in professional development and individuals in clinical audit.
- To ensure that the PCD works within the Code of Professional Conduct and competencies according to the GDC curricula.

Further Reading

British Dental Association. Contract of Employment for Dental Hygienists. Available to members of the British Dental Association from 64 Wimpole Street, London W1G 8YS.

Inland Revenue. Employed or Self Employed. London: Inland Revenue Business Services IRS6, 1999.

General Dental Council. The Rolls of Dental Auxiliaries and Dentists Register (updated annually). London: General Dental Council.

Hillam D. A survey of hygienists qualifying from the Liverpool School of Dental Hygiene 1977–1998. Br Dent J 2000;188:150–153.

Singh A. Employee or self-employed. Dent Health 1995;34:5–7.

International English Language Testing System. Cambridge: University of Cambridge Local Examinations Syndicate, 1997–2003.

Chapter 3
Working Together

Aim

This chapter aims to guide the practitioner through their role as the team leader and how they can effectively utilise the dental hygienist in the non-surgical management of periodontal diseases.

Outcome

Having read this chapter the practitioner should be able to rationalise the key roles of himself or herself (Fig 3-1), the specialist periodontist, the dental hygienist and the patient in achieving a successful therapeutic outcome, and the factors influencing this such as:

- the opportunistic aggressive nature of the disease
- complicating systemic and local risk factors (see Chapple and Gilbert 2002)
- patient understanding and compliance
- operator expertise and time management
- limiting socioeconomic factors
- rigour of the supportive care (maintenance) programme.

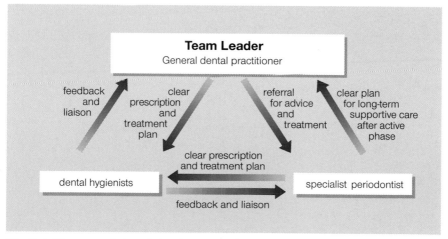

Fig 3-1 The general dental practitioner as the team leader.

Introduction

The first step in successful management of periodontal disease is to establish a diagnosis and formulate an appropriate treatment plan. This is the dentist's legal responsibility. The evidence for recording the prevalence of periodontal diseases in patients managed in general dental practice in the UK is currently very disappointing. In a study by Morgan in 2001, who examined 464 clinical records, only 20% included periodontal screening and only 1.5% (7 cases) had some form of periodontal charting − yet the cost of periodontal care to the National Health Service per annum is over £174 million (DPB website 2002). Does this imply that:

- Treatment is carried out without a diagnosis?
- Screening is not routinely performed in practice?
- Screening and periodontal examination are not recorded in practice?

These data suggest that current expenditure on periodontal therapy under the NHS service regulations may not be justified by the evidence documented in the clinical notes.

Only by screening and recording each and every patient at every examination and recall appointment will the periodontal needs of the population be identified and treatment targeted at patients of "high risk". It is inappropriate to prescribe for the patient a "routine scale and polish" every six months. The patient requires an individual care plan specifically to target sites of recurrent disease. The background to this concept is clearly outlined in the first book of this series (Chapple and Gilbert 2002).

Where there is no evidence of disease then no treatment is required. This may reflect on the entire mouth or individual teeth. The concept of selective scaling and selective root surface debridement (RSD) according to need must be established. This shift of emphasis must be explained to the patient (Chapter 5).

The practitioner must also be mindful of potential litigation. Currently, claims for failure to diagnose and treat periodontal disease amount to 4% of total claims, according to the Dental Defence Union (2001–2002). The number of claims is increasing, as is the average cost of settlement by defence organisations. Patients who have lost their natural dentition through proven negligence on the part of a practitioner now expect settlements to cover the provision of implants and their superstructures at enormous cost to the defence agencies and thus to the profession.

24

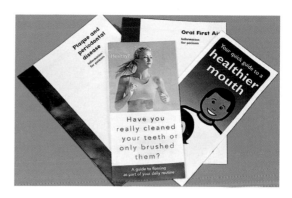

Fig 3-2 Patient information leaflets.

There is legal recognition of "the chance for a chance". It is not good practice for the practitioner to assume that the patient is not interested in treatment because their oral hygiene has been neglected previously. All treatment options should be discussed. If the patient chooses not to follow the advice they should be informed of the potential consequences and a record of the discussion made in the patient's clinical notes. It is good practice to utilise "practice produced" patient information leaflets. These may be given to the patient as supplementary information and evidence of this fact should be recorded in the clinical notes (Fig 3-2).

The Periodontal Treatment Plan and Referral to a Dental Hygienist

Details of the basic periodontal examination (BPE) and a comprehensive account of the initial screening visit is covered in the first book of this series (Chapple and Gilbert 2002). Following the BPE screen, any sextant coding 4 or 4★ will require detailed recording of probing pocket depths. Recording of bleeding on blunt probing also forms part of the clinical assessment. Good quality radiographs to assess the degree and pattern of bone loss are also essential (see Chapple and Gilbert 2002). It is the responsibility of the dentist to inform the patient of the diagnosis and prognosis and discuss all treatment options. Where disease is advanced this may include extractions and eventual prosthetic replacement. If the documentation of potential outcomes is robust (i.e. percentage of bone loss is recorded), it not only avoids potential litigation but it also provides valuable information for other team members. The dental hygienist should have the radiographs on view when treating the patient. Patients frequently ask the hygienist questions regarding the prognosis of their dentition. It is not within the remit of the hygien-

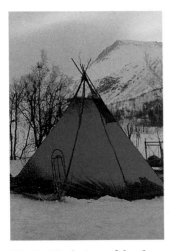

Fig 3-3 Isolation of the dental hygienist.

ist to make such statements, but if outcomes are written in the care plan, the hygienist can endorse and support the decisions of the prescribing dentist. This consolidates the team approach.

Communication Within the Team

A common concern expressed by dental hygienists working in general dental practice is that they feel isolated (Fig 3-3). Whilst the nature of their clinical work will always be within the legal framework, it is helpful for them to understand the holistic management of the patient, i.e. where the care they are providing juxtaposes with the care that other clinicians are providing. This helps the hygienist focus the patient on longer-term goals.

Good communication is therefore important, both to provide fulfilment to the staff in the workplace and to avoid errors and ambiguity in the prescribing process.

Accurate objective records of the patient's periodontal status at the onset of therapy and throughout treatment are essential. This is achieved by using recognised charts and indices. Indices are vital for:

- the education of the patient and for individual target setting
- information for clinicians to determine entry into more complex therapies
- medicolegal purposes.

Terms such as "good", "fair", or "poor" relating to the patient's plaque control are not acceptable as they are not objective methods of expressing factual information between professionals. Plaque accumulation and marginal (immediate) bleeding should be recorded using a reproducible scoring system (see Chapple and Gilbert 2002). The location of plaque deposits can only be scored accurately if the plaque is visible to the clinician. The use of a disclosing dye is therefore recommended (Fig 3-4).

There are advantages and disadvantages with the use of various indices. Whichever is selected should be uniformly used by all clinicians in the practice to facilitate case discussion and record transfer. History of tobacco use

26

by the patient should also be recorded in the notes at the initial stage, along with any advice given.

The Dentist as a Prescriber of Treatment

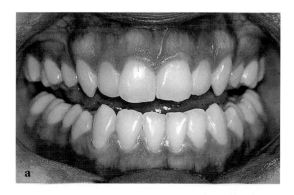

When presenting the treatment plan to the patient, care should be taken to give equal emphasis to the importance of all aspects of oral health care. For example, phrases such as "you *just* need a scale" or "only a quick clean up with the hygienist" imply lesser importance of periodontal health, relative to restorative needs. They also undermine the skills of the hygienist and may give the patient the impression that deposit removal is

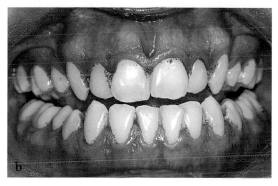

Fig 3-4 The use of disclosing dye to visualise plaque.

only for improvement in aesthetics. At the initial appointment the practitioner should discuss the involvement of the hygienist in the care plan and advise the patient of the advantages of referral. Case discussion between clinicians in the presence of the patient is very worthwhile. This establishes a "trialogue" in which the patient becomes informed and involved in their care plan (Fig 3-5). In particular, this is helpful at the initial appointment when the treatment plan is being discussed with the patient. If the dentist introduces the dental hygienist to the patient at this stage, it may help to overcome the patient's initial reluctance to see another clinician. This continuity may help to foster the professional relationship that is so important for patient motivation. The patient needs:
- information on the skills and role of the hygienist
- an estimate of the time commitment
- an estimate of the financial commitment
- information on when they will see the dentist for reassessment

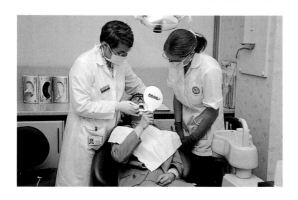

Fig 3-5 Including the patient in the care plan.

- a realistic understanding of treatment outcomes
- the side effects of treatment, especially recession and sensitivity.

The hygienist needs:
- diagnostic information
- a clearly stated treatment plan (It is a legal requirement that the prescription is in writing and signed and dated by the practitioner to cover a maximum 12-month period.)
- support from the referrer, as and when required.

The clinical records will serve as the main means of communication between the team leader and the PCD. The practitioner may like to consider the use of a pro forma. This method helps the clinician to focus on the needs of the patient. It avoids time-consuming writing of scripts and it is helpful to indicate the time frame of treatment in terms of numbers of visits, or time recommended for completion of a specific phase of management. A sample pro forma, a periodontal pocket chart, a plaque score chart and a bleeding score chart are illustrated in Figs 3-6 to 3-8.

Whilst pro formas help avoid unacceptable prescribing (Box 3-1), they suffer from the inevitable consequence of automatic behaviour patterns. The practitioner must remember to "think outside the box" and separately document individual patient data that does not appear on the pro forma. This can be achieved by writing on top of the pro forma.

Hygienist Prescription *(please tick)*

Staff Hygienist ☐

Patient's name/Bar code

Date ....

School of Hygiene:

Senior ☐

Relevant Medical History
(see medical history sheet) ☐

Junior ☐

Diagnosis [   ]

BPE ┼┼

Hygiene Phase Therapy   Full mouth ☐   Localised ☐
(specify area)

Disclose ☐   Toothbrushing ☐
Modified Bass   Toothbrushing
other (specify) ....

Floss/Tape ☐   Mini-interproximal ☐
Superfloss   brush   Interspace brush
(specify area) ┼┼

Charting   Pre-treatment ☐   & Post-treatment ☐

Full mouth ☐   Localised ☐
(specify area)

Plaque score ☐   Pocket charting ☐   BOP ☐   Mobility ☐

Scaling   Full mouth ☐   Localised ☐
(specify area)

Gross scale ☐   Fine scale ☐

Root Planing   All sites ≥ 5mm ☐

(under LA if required) ☐

Number of visits ☐   More if ☐
needed (tick)

Antibiotic Prophylaxis required (specify) ....

Topical fluoride application (specify) ....

Dietary analysis/advice ....

Review [Months]   With
(print/stamp) [   ]

Referred by ....
(print/stamp)

Signature of ....
referring clinician

Fig 3-6 An example of prescription pro forma (from a teaching hospital) for referral to the dental hygienist.

29

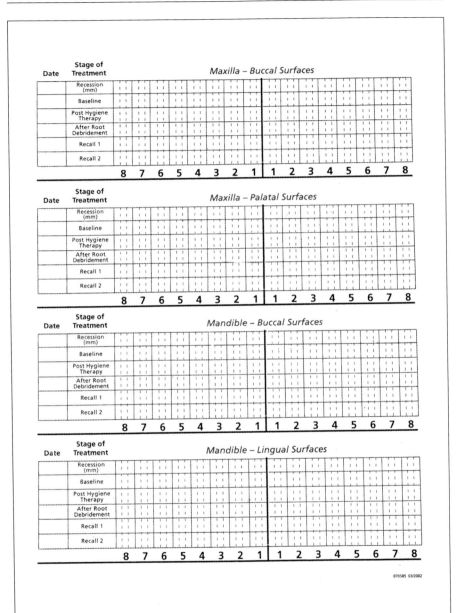

Fig 3-7 A periodontal pocket chart.

Full Mouth Periodontal Assessment

Patient's Name: _____   Registration Number: _____

Date:_____   Operator: _____

Plaque Score

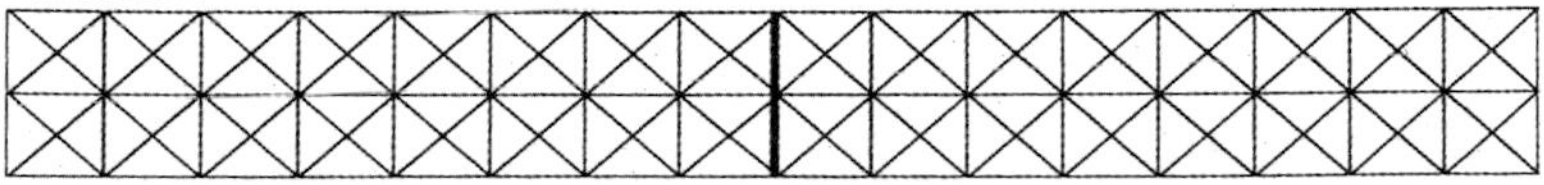

Total Score: _____   Plaque Surface % : _____
Plaque Free Surface % : _____

Bleeding Score

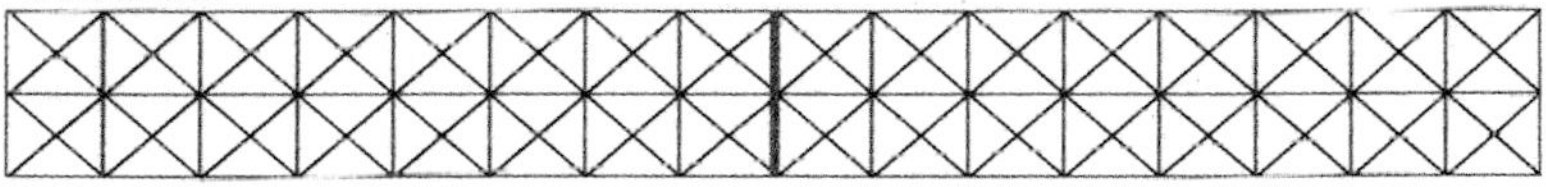

Total Score: _____   Bleeding %: _____

Date:_____   Operator: _____

Plaque Score

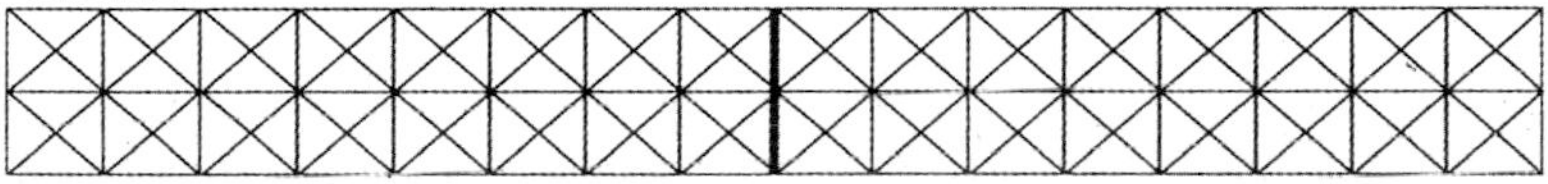

Total Score: _____   Plaque Surface % : _____
Plaque Free Surface % : _____

Bleeding Score

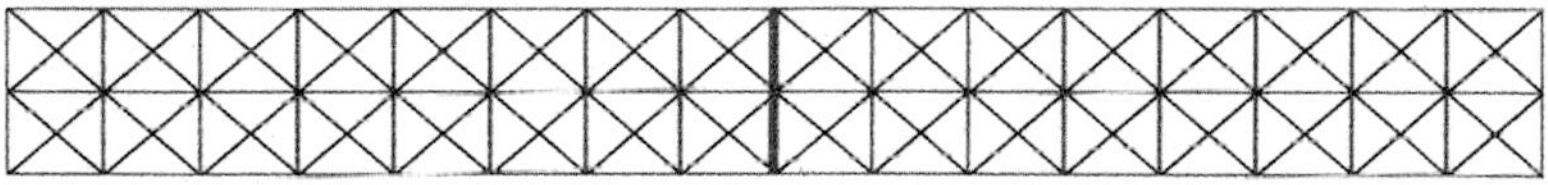

Total Score: _____   Bleeding %: _____

Date:_____   Operator: _____

Plaque Score

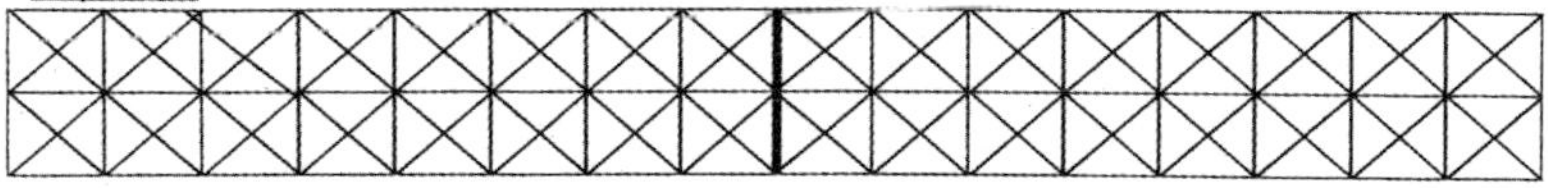

Total Score: _____   Plaque Surface % : _____
Plaque Free Surface % : _____

Bleeding Score

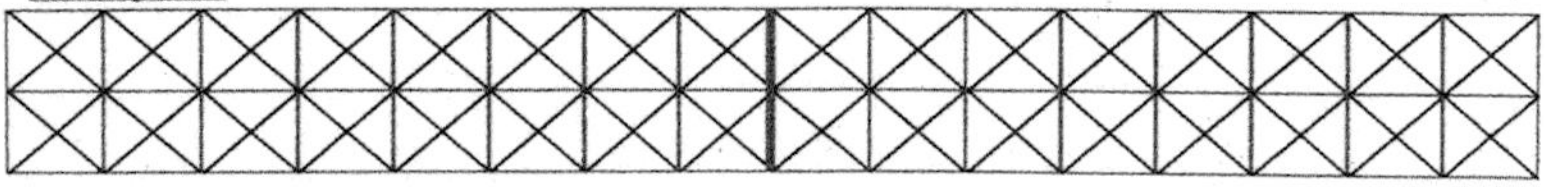

Total Score: _____   Bleeding %: _____

Fig 3-8 A plaque and bleeding score chart.

Box 3-1

> **Examples of unacceptable prescriptions**
> *Hygienist please see and treat*
> *Scp x1 (or S&P)*
> *Item 10a please*
> *OH poor, ref. Hygienist*

None of those "prescriptions" gives any indication of the nature or the severity of periodontal disease and would be indefensible medicolegally.

Whilst considering the treatment to be prescribed it may be more economic of the practitioner's time to designate the recording of base line indices, including probing depths to the hygienist. However, the practitioner must perform the BPE and report on the radiographs (see Chapple and Gilbert 2002). The post-therapy detailed charting should also be performed by the practitioner, to enable them to "get a feel" for the requirements of the second phase of therapy for the individual patient.

Dental hygienists are trained to record:
• periodontal probing depths
• recession
• clinical attachment levels
• mobility
• furcation involvement
• full mouth bleeding (dichotomously)
• full mouth plaque deposits (dichotomously)
• drifting (by measurement, study models)
• occlusion (static and dynamic).

Dental hygienists are trained to advise and educate on:
• dietary habits (caries and erosion control)
• smoking cessation
• oral cleaning of hard and soft tissues, implants and prostheses
• why the patient is a special case, specifically "at risk" of periodontitis.
The patient must feel that they have a unique problem which requires oral hygiene practices different from their peers and family (rather like the dia-

betic patient who needs to monitor what they eat and their blood glucose levels, the patient with periodontitis needs to monitor plaque levels and how they control them).

Of particular help in the prescription is guidance on the number of appointments for treatment with the hygienist and an indication of when review appointments with the dentist should be expected. This is also necessary to avoid open-ended prescriptions. It is illegal to prescribe for longer than 12 months. Without a review date, there is no indication of an end-point to evaluate the treatment.

It is a relatively common practice for the patient at a recall appointment to see the dental hygienist first for scaling and then see the dentist for the hard tissue examination. This is unacceptable practice because the hygienist is carrying out treatment on a "prescription", which is six months old! Whilst this is not "illegal" the prescription does not carry a current diagnosis and therefore will not address the current treatment needs of the patient. Furthermore, the prescriber will not be assessing the current medical history, and will be unable to perform accurate periodontal probing after periodontal intervention by the hygienist.

Dental hygienists require continuous support from their prescribing dentist in making decisions regarding the patient's overall care and, in particular, if the patient requires specialist periodontal care. If the patient has aggressive periodontitis, it is helpful to designate a time frame for appointments and whether liaison will be required regarding the administration of systemic antibiotics. Therefore, based on the practitioner's diagnosis, and the hygienist's clinical expertise, valuable clinical time can be appropriately targeted at the "at risk" patients with appointments scheduled accordingly. Patients in low risk categories do not require the same degree of intensive therapy, and it is the dentist's responsibility to indicate this by the number and frequency of visits on the prescription.

If the patient is medically compromised, it is the dentist's responsibility to ensure that care during the hygienist's phase of management is appropriate. The dentist should indicate if antibiotic prophylaxis is required and prescribe it for the patient; they should organise any adjustment of anticoagulant therapy; and prescribe specific local analgesic agents, if required.

If two kinds of treatment can be combined to conserve the administration of prophylactic antibiotics, then it is the dentist's responsibility to organise this – for example, scaling and an extraction in one appointment session. It is, however, the dental hygienist's responsibility to check the medical history at every visit and report any changes to the dentist.

Summary of the role of the dental practitioner as the team leader

The general dental practitioner is responsible for:
- Diagnosis.
- Treatment planning.
- Delegation to PCDs.
- The patients overall care plan.
- Quality control and audit.

Guidelines for prescribing to the dental hygienist are summarised in Box 3-2.

Box 3-2

> *Detailed written instructions (a pro forma may help).*
>
> *Indication as to the number of visits for initial therapy.*
>
> *Use of local analgesia.*
>
> *Organisation of antibiotic prophylaxis and management of anticoagulant therapy.*
>
> *Review date with the dentist.*

The Role of the Dental Hygienist

First phase of treatment

In the initial "oral hygiene" phase of treatment, the dental hygienist:
- Educates the patient as to the cause of disease and its management, and motivates the patient to bring about effective changes.
- Assists the patient in managing the cause-related aspect of their care, e.g. plaque control and smoking cessation counselling (Chapter 5).
- Monitors the response to therapy by recording the plaque and bleeding scores and offers appropriate individual oral hygiene advice and encouragement to maintain effective plaque control.
- Meticulously removes supra- and subgingival deposits and performs subgingival debridement to remove infected and necrotic cementum. The latter is a demanding clinical task that requires adequate time-allocation and use of appropriate subgingival instruments (see third book of the present series – *Successful Periodontal Therapy: A Non-Surgical Approach*).

On completion of this initial hygiene phase it is recommended to delay periodontal probing and future therapy for a period of 6 to 12 weeks to allow:
- resolution of inflammation within the marginal tissues
- recession and hence reduction in probing pocket depths
- remodelling of connective tissues within the gingival cuff (tightening of cuff)
- re-establishment of a non-pathogenic subgingival microflora.

And to assess:
- plaque control compliance
- response to smoking cessation advice, if appropriate.

The protocol for the transition from the initial phase to the corrective phase of therapy will depend upon the individual practice. In formulating this protocol, the practitioner needs to consider the skill and experience of the hygienist with whom they are working.

Investment in skills development and equipment is essential for success (Chapter 4). The practitioner has an obligation as an employer in this regard to ensure that the hygienist is encouraged to attend appropriate hands-on courses, and to provide the necessary equipment in the practice.

Review with the dentist
A review with the prescribing dentist will determine the extent of the patient's compliance with plaque control and smoking cessation; where "active" periodontal sites are located; and whether there are any plaque retention factors that could be addressed at this stage of therapy. The evidence that will guide the practitioner to form a revised treatment plan may be obtained from the monitoring charts, the clinical notes and the radiographs. The "subject-based", "tooth-based", and "site-based" risk assessments are outlined in the first book of this series.

Of particular significance are:
- Any change in the patient's medical history.
- The full mouth bleeding and plaque scores (Fig 3-9).
- The detailed pocket chart at the end of the initial phase of therapy to be compared with the base line chart (Fig 3-10).
- Record of patient attendance.
- Record of smoking habits (if appropriate).
- Any defective restorations.

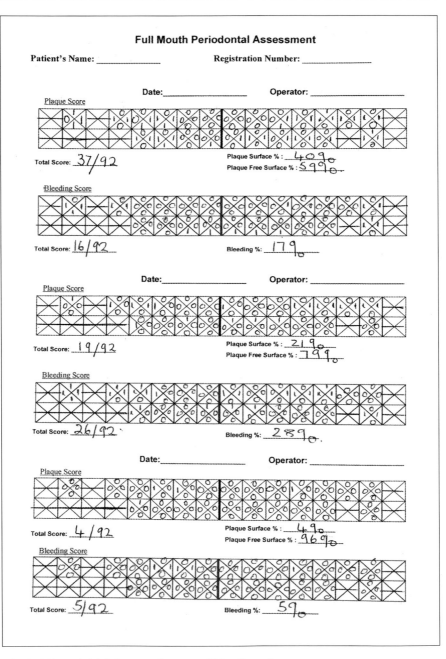

Fig 3-9 Post-initial therapy plaque and bleeding chart.

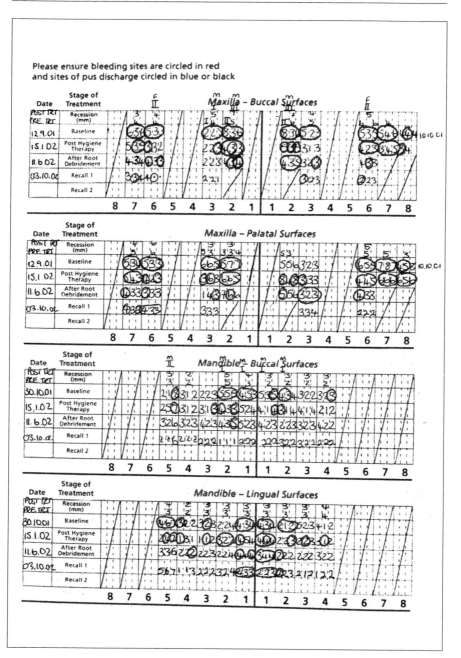

Fig 3-10 A pocket chart on completion of the initial phase of therapy.

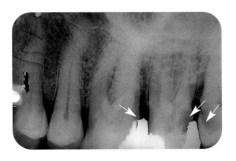

Fig 3-11 An overhanging restoration should be replaced at the completion of the initial phase of therapy and active caries removed during the initial phase.

From this the practitioner can determine which plaque retention factors could be eliminated at this stage to enhance plaque removal and aid healing. Overhanging or defective restorations (Fig 3-11) could be renewed and defective crowns could be replaced with laboratory-constructed crowns with good marginal adaptation and emergence profiles. Decisions concerning other factors which may affect disease recurrence, for example mucosal factors such as a high fraenal attachment, overcrowding and denture replacement should be deferred until the periodontal tissues are stable.

Which sites require RSD?
The greatest risk of disease progression is in pockets with a probing depth ≥5 mm, which bleed on probing. This refers to bleeding from the base of the pocket, which is sometimes termed "delayed bleeding". It is helpful if these pockets are identified on the chart by using red ink to record the depth in millimetres. These sites can be debrided by the dental hygienist under local analgesia, following which the patient should be reviewed by the dentist, allowing a minimum of 6–12 weeks for the healing process.

Second phase of treatment
The GDP's revised or "phase 2" treatment plan to the hygienist should:
- Indicate areas where plaque control is inadequate and identify any site-specific risk factors, e.g. root grooves.
- Prescribe sites which are to be root debrided under local analgesia.
- Request a review appointment with the dentist 2–3 months after the final session of root debridement.

In non–responding sites the hygienist may, if prescribed, apply locally delivered antimicrobial agents as an adjunct to root surface debridement.

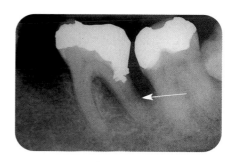

Fig 3-12 Root caries is a frequent sequela of managed periodontitis.

Supportive Periodontal Therapy

The dental hygienist may also play a key role in supportive periodontal (or maintenance) therapy. Many studies (e.g. Axelsson and Lindhe 1981, Ramfjord, *et al.* 1982) have demonstrated that treatment will fail if the patient is not reviewed frequently.

When does supportive therapy start?
Supportive therapy starts when the patient has learnt to reduce and maintain plaque levels to an extent that the host response does not lead to clinical signs of inflammation and the disease is no longer active/progressive. In advanced cases maintenance may not begin until 18 months or two years have elapsed since initial diagnosis. A further prescription to the dental hygienist is required, including guidance on the frequency of recall visits. The frequency will depend on the:

- host response (i.e. the individual patient's threshold for plaque accumulation)
- complexity of the dentition and oral musculature
- manual dexterity of the patient
- lifestyle factors (shift work, stress, etc.).

It is the dentist's responsibility to monitor diseases of the hard tissues. Root caries is a frequent sequela of managed periodontal diseases (Fig 3-12) and is often only detected radiographically. The commencement of the maintenance phase is also the appropriate time in the overall care plan to discuss tooth replacement and any concerns regarding recession.

Case Discussion

The team will strengthen as a result of case discussion throughout the various stages of treatment. Shared successful and unsuccessful outcomes can

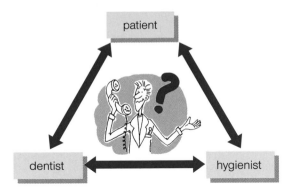

Fig 3-13 Communication of the message.

become the basis for peer review, education and clinical audit. This, in turn, may lead to a review of practice protocols. To formalise this process a case study presented at a practice meeting will inform other team members. If personnel other than the dentist are invited in rotation to lead the presentation it builds on the individual involvement within the team.

Key points of clinical relevance (Fig 3-13)

The dentist's responsibilities:
- To explane the diagnosis and prognosis in terms that the patient can understand.
- To maintain accurate written and radiographic records.
- To describe the role of the dental hygienist to the patient
- To make clear the time and financial commitment to the patient.
- To have good written and oral communication with the dental hygienist.
- To arrange regular review appointments.

The hygienist's responsibilities:
- To educate, motivate and counsel the patient.
- Effectively to remove deposits.
- To liaise with the directing clinician when necessary.

Further Reading

Axelsson P, Lindhe J. The significance of maintenance care in the treatment of peri-odontal disease. J Clin Periodontol 1981;8:281–295.

Chapple ILC, Gilbert AD. Understanding Periodontal Diseases: Assessment and Diagnostic Procedures in Practice. London: Quintessence, 2002.

Dental Defence Union. Claims Notified to the Dental Defence Union from UK GDP Members 2001–2002. London: MDU, 2002.

Dental Practice Board. Non-surgical periodontal NHS treatment to September 2002 in England and Wales over 18 and under 18 years. www.dpb.nhs.uk/ddonline/digest_result.cfm/.

Morgan RG. Quality evaluation of clinical records of a group of general dental prac-titioner entering a quality assurance programme. Br Dent J 2001;191:436–441.

Ramfjord SP, Morrison EC, Bergett FG, Nissle RR, Shick RA, Zann GJ, Knowles JW. Oral hygiene and maintenance of periodontal support. J Periodontol 1982;53:26–30.

Chapter 4
Selecting Surgery Equipment for the Dental Hygienist

Aim

The aim of this chapter is to highlight the specific surgery requirements for a dental hygienist to manage periodontal disease efficiently and effectively.

Outcome

Having read this chapter, clinicians will have a source of reference for the selection of instruments and equipment recommended for the dental hygienist.

The Decision-Making Process

Before deciding on the requirements for a surgery, it is important to gather and collate information from various sources (Fig 4-1).

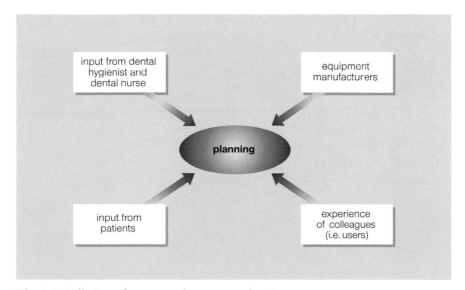

Fig 4-1 Collation of resources for surgery planning.

The Surgery Layout and Equipment

It is not the remit of this book to include details of general dental equipment common to all surgeries, but rather to focus on the specific requirements of dental hygienists. Some of these may be similar to those of a dentist's surgery but other requirements differ.

The hygienist requires as much operative space as the dentist and the equipment and layout should give a similar impression to the patient to when they enter the dentist's surgery. Patients with periodontal disease are likely to visit the hygienist more often than the dentist. It is therefore important to create an environment of comfort and relaxation compatible with universal cross-infection control procedures. If the hygienist has "second-hand" equipment in a small room, it is worth reflecting on the image this may portray to the patient (Fig 4-2).

A key priority in surgery planning is ergonomics. Dental clinicians suffer from occupational musculoskeletal problems and hygienists are no exception. According to MacDonald and colleagues (1988), approximately 29% of hygienists suffer from carpal tunnel syndrome and other associated upper body neuropathies. There are several risk factors contributing to the occupational component of this syndrome (Box 4-1). The utilisation of the working space, the equipment, and choice of the instruments are essential considerations in the preventive strategies for a condition which is painful and debilitating or may, in some cases, lead to forced early retirement.

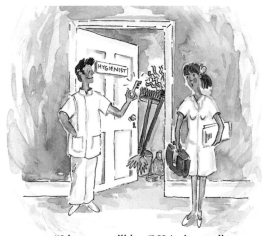

"I hope you'll be OK in here..."

Fig 4-2 "Welcome to the broom cupboard."

Box 4-1

Major Risk Factors in Carpal Tunnel Syndrome

Operator position

Force needed to grasp instrument handles

Mechanical stress from power leads and cords

Vibration from ultrasonics

Temperature of surgery and hand washing water

Posture

Dental hygienists work from the 12 o'clock to the 8 o'clock chair positions. For a right-handed operator, treatment of the lower anterior, lower right posterior, upper anterior and upper right posterior sextants is frequently conducted with the patient semi-supine and the hygienist facing the patient (Fig 4-3). This positioning enables the operator to work by direct vision and to keep the lower back upright and the wrist in the neutral position. Wrist flexion increases compression in the carpal tunnel by 200%. In order to achieve the optimal position there must be sufficient space for the operator's chair to be manoeuvred between the dental chair and the fixed cabinetry.

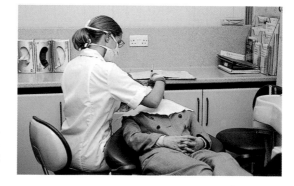

Fig 4-3 Positioning of both patient and operator is important in maintaining good posture.

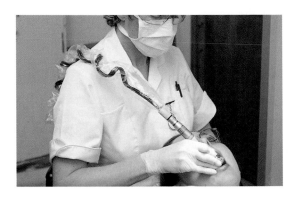

Fig 4-4 Support of the hand piece cord reduces force on the wrist.

Force

Handpieces attached to curled cords tend to exert greater force on the wrist. This design should preferably be avoided, but if they are already installed then the hygienist can support the cord to minimise the force (Fig 4-4).

Similarly, with hand instruments, grasping and forceful exertion during scaling may lead to symptoms. This can be avoided by using ergonomically designed, silicone covered lightweight instruments. Thin hexagonal shaped handles require more force and pushing to secure them in the fingers (Figs 4-5 and 4-6). This also contributes to mechanical stress. Vibration damage to the small blood vessels occurs at 20–80 Hz. Whilst the ultrasonic scaler is an essential part of the hygienist's equipment, it is useful to plan appointments so that its use is not continuous.

Temperature

Low temperature constricts the blood flow and accentuates the symptoms of nerve-end compression. The ambient temperature should be around 25 °C.

Radiographic Equipment

Dental hygienists who have undertaken the IR(ME)R2000 regulations training are permitted to take radiographs prescribed by the dentist. If x-ray equipment is installed in their surgery, or at a designated x-ray workstation, this will enable dental hygienists optimally to utilise their skills. However, if the equipment is solely in the dentist's surgery they are less likely to be called upon to take radiographs because of the economic use of surgery time.

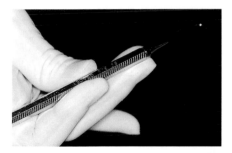

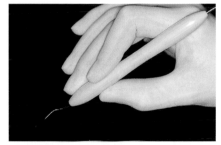

Fig 4-5 Hexagonal shaped handles are pinched to ensure a sound grip.

Fig 4-6 An ergonomically designed silicone handle is held lightly.

This will lead to the hygienist becoming de-skilled and loosing confidence in taking radiographs.

Equipment for Patient Education

As discussed in Chapter 3, the dental hygienist has a vital role to play in informing the patient about the nature of the disease in their mouth. The education may be personalised by the use of intraoral cameras and phase-contrast microscopy which allows the hygienist to demonstrate plaque organisms magnified × 1000 (Fig 4-7). This is an excellent motivating tool as comparative samples can be taken at subsequent appointments to review plaque control.

Equipment for Scaling and Root Debridement

The reader is referred to Fig 4-8 for the equipment and instruments recommended for safe, effective clinical practice.

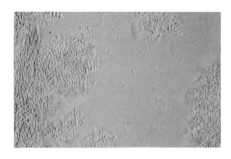

Fig 4-7 Phase-contrast microscopy to demonstrate plaque morphotypes (× 1000).

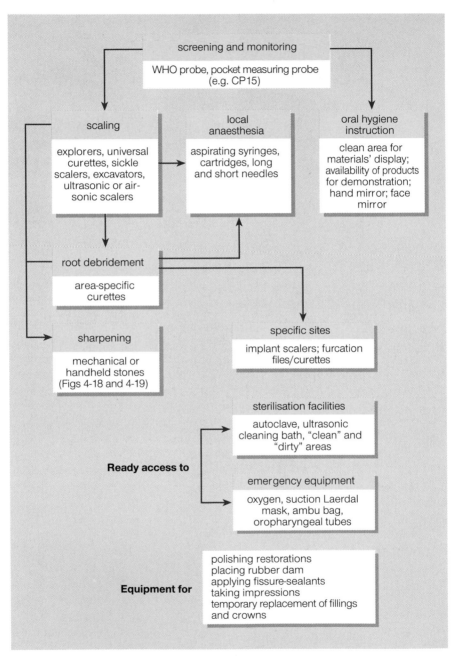

Fig 4-8 Specific equipment for the dental hygienist's surgery.

Fig 4-9 WHO probe.

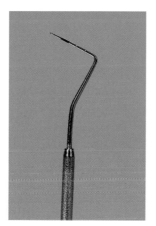
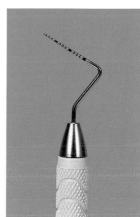

Fig 4-10 Periodontal measuring probe.

Screening

The WHO probe (Fig 4-9) is essential for Basic Periodontal Examinaton screening. Its ball end is also suitable for establishing bleeding on probing.

Monitoring

The periodontal measuring probe, usually with graduations up to 15 mm, is essential for measuring probing pocket depths (Fig 4-10).

It may also be used for measuring recession thus providing an indication of true attachment loss. The WHO probe cannot be used for longitudinal assessment as the bands representing the codes merely distinguish between moderate and advanced disease. "Measuring" becomes a "guesstimate". Disclosing dye is necessary for recording the presence of plaque.

Scaling

The removal of plaque and calculus from the root surface requires the following:
1. Mechanical scalers
   Ultrasonic magnetostrictive scalers
   These operate at 20–40 KHz and work by mechanical chipping, cavitation and acoustic microstreaming. Schroedar valves are necessary for installation. Studies by Chapple *et al.* (1992, 1995) demonstrated that the half-power mode was as effective as the full-power mode and less likely

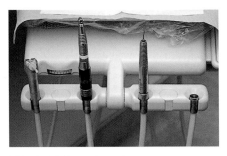

Fig 4-11 A sonic scaler.

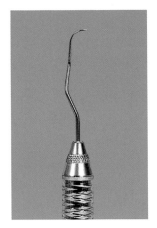

Fig 4-12 The ODU periodontal explorer (Hu Friedy, Chicago).

to cause root surface damage, and that there was no efficacy gain (over water) by using chlorhexidine, for irrigation. Caution is necessary with patients who have the older types of pacemaker fitted. Piezo-electric scalers are an alternative ultrasonic scaler. The mode of action is via a quartz crystal in the hand piece which deforms when subjected to alternating voltages. The deformation drives the tip oscillation.

Sonic scalers
These operate at <20 KHz and are driven by compressed air from the dental unit (Fig 4-11). They are damped down by contact of the tip with the tooth, but they can be used on patients with older pacemakers.

2. High volume aspiration
3. Nursing assistance
4. Hand instruments
   - universal curettes which cut on both sides of the tip and are useful for heavy deposits of subgingival calculus
   - sickle scalers for supragingival deposits
   - excavators
5. Hand pieces, rubber cups, points and brushes. The screw insertion is recommended rather than the latch grip attachments. This is because the prophylaxis paste will encourage wear and tear of the bearings.

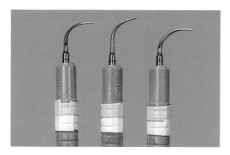
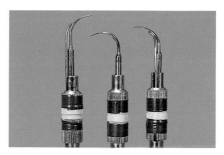

Fig 4-13 The slimline cavitron tips (Densply, Weybridge, Surrey) with focused spray.

Fig 4-14 External water delivery Cavitron tips of limited use. Entry into pockets > 7mm is impossible.

Root surface debridement

Root surface debridement requires thorough instrumentation of the root surface and removal of endotoxin-associated cementum. The dental hygienist will perform this as a closed procedure. It is difficult to perform and requires careful identification of the deposits followed by meticulous removal. Careful technique will also avoid both root surface and soft tissue trauma. In order to aim for a favourable healing response, the lipopolysaccharide (endotoxin) associated with the surface (10–15%) of cementum must be removed. Appropriate instruments include:

1. The Old Dominican University (ODU) explorer. This is used prior to root debridement to detect subgingival deposits and afterwards to ensure deposits have been removed. It has a long flexible shank and requires a light pressure for tactile sensation. It is far superior to the WHO probe for detection of deposits (Fig 4-12).
2. Curved furcation probe
3. Ultrasonic and sonic scaler tips for root debridement. The tips with the longer terminal shanks are required to reach towards the base of the pockets. The ultrasonic scaler tips are available as slim line tips with a focused spray (Fig 4-13). There are older models available with an external water delivery but use is limited as entry to pockets ≥7 mm is impossible due to obstruction by the water tube (Fig 4-14).
4. Hand instruments – Area-specific Gracey curettes. These are the hand instruments of choice for closed root debridement having long curved

flexible shanks and blades at 70° to the shank. The blades are contoured to the root surface and cut on one side and therefore are used at specific sites only. A suggested range of site-specific curettes for the hygienist is given in Box 4-2 and Fig 4-15. Hoes have straight shank ends and one point tooth contact. Some have tungsten carbide cutting blades which means that they cannot be sharpened in the surgery. These have been largely superseded by area-specific curettes.

Box 4-2

Area-specific Gracey Curettes

1/2 All surfaces of anterior teeth

7/8 Facial and lingual surfaces of premolars

9/10 Facial and lingual surfaces of molars

11/12 Mesial surfaces of posterior teeth

13/14 Distal surfaces of posterior teeth

15/16 Mesial surfaces of posterior teeth of difficult access

17/18 Distal Surfaces of posterior teeth of difficult access

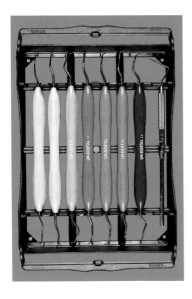

Fig 4-15 Area-specific Gracey curettes (LM Dental, Finland).

Fig 4-16 Furcation files.

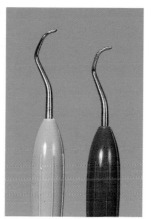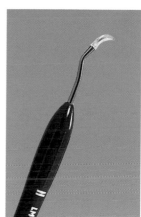

Fig 4-17 Scalers for cleaning implants.

Additional instruments for specific sites

These may include:

- Furcation files (Fig 4-16) and hoes.
- Mini area-specific curettes. These instruments have a blade diameter 50% of standard area-specific curettes and are useful in narrow deep pockets.
- Gold- or plastic-tipped scalers for implants(Fig 4-17).

Equipment for Local Anaesthesia

- Aspirating syringes.
- Long and short needles.
- Anaesthetic cartridges.
- Surface anaesthetic cream.
- A "sharps" bin.
- A separate cytotoxic waste bin (for anaesthetic cartridges).

Sharpening Equipment

Scaling instruments, apart from those specific for implants are manufactured from martensitic stainless steel. An instrument becomes dull during use because the tooth surface is harder than the metal of the instrument and particles are lost from the surface. To resharpen a scaling instrument, the material of the sharpening stone must be harder than the steel of the instrument. The reasons for sharpening scaling instruments are listed in Box 4-3.

Box 4-3

Reasons for sharpening scaling instruments

Decrease in operator time (fewer strokes are required)

Increase in the control of the instrument (greater precision is possible)

Decrease in risk of soft tissue trauma

Decreased operator fatigue

Reduction in burnishing of the calculus

Improve tactile sensitivity (a light grasp is possible)

The goals of sharpening

To produce a sharp edge

To preserve the instrument design and conserve the blades (manufacturers recommend that instruments be replaced when the blade has been reduced by 50%).

The requisites for sharpening

A stone (hand held or power driven)

A magnifying loupe

A plastic test stick

The hand–held stone may be natural material such as Arkansas or a ceramic material (Fig 4-18). This method requires knowledge of the instrument design, skill and patience! Electronic sharpening stones are an efficient and accurate method of sharpening instruments (Fig 4-19). There are, however, two major disadvantages compared to mechanical stones: the instruments must be sterile, therefore the machine cannot be used during an operative procedure; and they are expensive.

Domiciliary Visits

From time to time hygienists are required to leave the surgery environment and visit patients in their own or residential homes. It is a legal requirement that a third person is present. The ideal person is the dental nurse who is able to assist and advise during the treatment. A suggested list of equipment and

Fig 4-18 A hand-held sharpening kit.

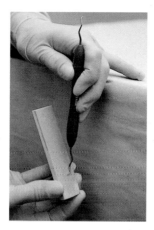
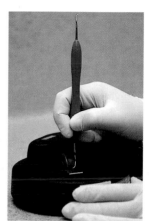

Fig 4-19 An electronic sharpening stone (LM Dental, Finland. El-Rondo from JS Davis).

Table 4-1 **Machine sharpening.**

Advantages	Disadvantages
• Quick • Straightforward to use • Precise adaptation of the instrument design; conserves the blades • Any member of the dental team can use the machine	• Only sterile instruments, can be sharpened and hand-held stones should also be available for sharpening during treatment • Relatively costly

materials for domiciliary visits is shown in Table 4-2. This equipment and materials can be packed in a plastic toolbox. In addition, the possession of car insurance for employment purposes is recommended.

Dental Nursing Support

It is desirable to provide designated nursing support to the dental hygienist for the following reasons:
• Cross-infection control.
• Recording of indices into the clinical notes requires a third person.
• Aspiration – the ultrasonic and air scalers create hazardous aerosols.
• Chaperone.
• Four-handed support – for patient comfort and safety, aspiration, fissure-sealant application, local anaesthetic, medical emergency.

Table 4-2 **Suggested kit for domiciliary visit by dental hygienist.**

Essentials	Portable equipment	Sterile instruments	Disposables	Medicaments
ID badge	Portable suction	Exam packs (1 extra)	Gloves	Mouthwash tablets
Clinical top (and spare)	Mobile unit and hand-pieces	Polishing packs	Masks	Vaseline™
Plastic aprons	Portable lamp	Scaling pack	Dappens pots	Toothpaste
Protective goggles	Sharps bin		Denture pots	Duraphat™ varnish
Pen and paper			Cups	Prophylaxis paste
Diary			Tongue depressors	Chlorhexidine gel and mouthwash
Appointment cards			Gauze (individually wrapped)	Toothbrushes
Record cards			Cotton wool rolls/ pledgets	Interdental brushes
NHS forms			Swabs	Floss and tape
Telephone number (contact)			Tissues	Disclosing tablets
Mobile phone			Baby wipes	Surface disinfectant
Torch			Rubbish bags	
Treatment sheet				

- Economy of time – during sterilisation, patient transference and development of radiographs.

With nursing support the dental hygienist will work more efficiently and reduce problems induced by poor posture.

When only the dental hygienist and patient are on the premises, it is essential that a second suitably qualified individual is present when the dental hygienist provides treatment. Usually this will be a qualified dental nurse.

Key Points of Clinical Relevance

- In order to utilise their full range of skills and to perform competently, the dental hygienist requires a comprehensive range of effective instruments and appropriate materials.
- The dental equipment and surgery design require the same high standards in planning and execution as that for the dentist's surgery.
- Cross-infection control and health and safety at work are top priorities in surgery design.
- Dental nursing support is essential.
- Consider the patients' impressions of all clinical environments.

Further Reading

Chapple ILC, Walmsley AD, Saxby M, Moscrop H. Effect of instrument power setting during ultrasonic scaling upon treatment outcome. J Periodontol 1995;66:756–760.

Chapple ILC, Walmsley AD, Saxby M, Moscrop H. Effect of subgingival irrigation with chlorhexidine during ultrasonic scaling. J Periodontol 1992;63:812–816.

MacDonald G, Robinson HM, Erickson JA. Carpal tunnel syndrome among California dental hygienists. Dent Hygienist 1988;62:323–328.

Chapter 5
Prevention of Oral Disease I: Periodontal Disease

Aim

This aim of this chapter is to guide the team through the promotion of effective oral hygiene and smoking cessation advice for the *individual* patient.

Outcome

The team members should have an understanding of the suggested methods of delivery of oral health messages to prevent diseases of the supporting tissues and the oral mucosa.

Oral Hygiene Instruction

Successful general dental practices have a co-ordinated team approach to the prevention of periodontal diseases. To achieve success consideration must be given to effective patient education and consistent long-term patient motivation.

Education

The more often oral health messages are transmitted to the patient utilising different forms of media, the more likely a positive response. First, the patient must accept that the advice applies to them as an individual and then they must commit themselves to achieving positive outcomes. From the outset the patient must recognise that they have a disease of the supporting tissues of their teeth, induced by microbial plaque and modified by their host response, that many others do not have. The education process commences with the dentist at diagnosis and is reinforced by the hygienist. It is strengthened by the nursing and reception staff, especially if they are responsible for advice on and selling of oral hygiene products. Human beings forget health messages, or do not identify with them. Reinforcement is therefore required at every visit and, in particular, at a recall appointment.

To be effective the patient requires consistent advice from the staff. In order to achieve this, practice policies should be discussed at team meetings. This may include a policy on which oral health products to offer for sale, or co-ordination of smoking cessation advice.

Motivation

According to the "expectancy value" theory of motivation, if a patient is to engage in an activity then they must value the outcome and expect success in achieving it. The impact of value and expectancy is multiplied. It is not simply additive; both factors need to be present. If either value or expectancy is absent then the motivated activity will not occur. The expectancy value theory is particularly relevant in the early stages of learning, i.e. when a patient first learns of the diagnosis of periodontal disease. The entire team has a key role to play in the value of addressing lifestyle changes and encouraging positive outcomes when these changes are acted upon.

Products in Practice

It is advisable to appoint a co-ordinator who regularly updates the products and consults with clinicians regarding specific requirements. In practices with an input from visiting specialists, the products may range from maintenance of implants to fixed orthodontic appliances. Chemical plaque control and dentifrices should also be available with the emphasis being on proven efficacy in independent randomised clinical trials. Representatives can be very persuasive, but must be able to provide evidence if requested to substantiate their claims. Recommended oral hygiene products should be:

• individualised
• readily available
• effective
• good value for money
• easy to use.

Individual Instruction

Oral hygiene aids must be individualised. It may be stating the obvious but each patient's mouth is unique – in shape, size, dentition and musculature. Add to this the varying degrees of true and false pocketing, complex restorations, crowding of teeth, a hypersensitive gag reflex, dentures, and very different host responses, and plaque control becomes extremely complex!

Instructions to the patient, who may not be manually dextrous, or who has conflicting priorities in life, require effort, time and patience on the part of the clinician. They involve reinforcement over several visits, beginning with basic tooth brushing technique and progressing onto interdental cleaning once the mouth "map" has been imprinted in the patient's thinking.

The process includes breaking the cycle of unconscious actions carried out ineffectively. For some patients these processes may have been in place for over 50 years. These have to be replaced with new techniques, which at first will be consciously undertaken but later will become unconscious activities again. The "ladder of competence" paradigm used by teachers is relevant here (Fig 5-1).

Patients with periodontal disease have by definition an inappropriate host response to the microbial biofilm. In order to maintain health, they have to be highly efficient at plaque control. Furthermore, this exercise has no definitive time frame; it requires daily commitment for life!

Demonstration of plaque control has therefore to be on a one-to-one basis. It has to be given by a clinician who is legally permitted to place their hands inside a patient's mouth and who has an understanding of the patient's oral disease status, medical status and plaque retention factors. It does not necessarily have to be taught in the dental chair, but this is preferable for several reasons.

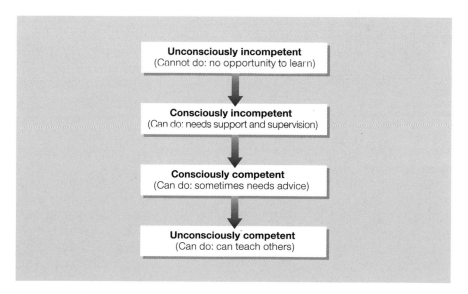

Fig 5-1 Ladder of competence.

The chair is manoeuvrable and has a head rest – this allows access to demonstrate difficult sites. There is a light source for good illumination of posterior sites. There will be a mouth mirror and a blunt probe available to aid education. There is a bowl for expectoration. Cross-infection control must be maintained.

Adults tend to be embarrassed by a demonstration on oral hygiene and, in particular, by having to practise it in front of others. To respect privacy, if a preventive unit is to be used it is advisable only to have one adult at a time. Children, on the other hand, have fewer oral complications, particularly the younger age groups with only the primary dentition to maintain. They usually require toothbrush instruction only and enjoy the company of other children. They may be instructed in a preventive dental unit environment with a trained oral health educator. For older children requiring interdental cleaning instructions and maintenance of fixed appliances, the more personal approach for adults should be followed.

How to give the advice

Broadly speaking, people can retain about seven pieces of information at any one time (Fig 5-2). If some of this information is visual and some linguistic, the total increases.

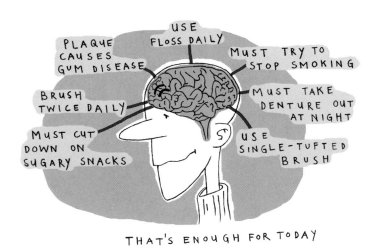

Fig 5-2 "My brain is about to burst."

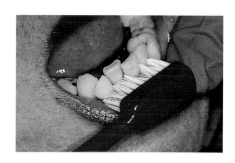

Fig 5-3 Identification of the individual problems.

If the patient hears the health message only, 20% of the information will be retained. If they see the message in a visual form, 50% of the information is retained. If the instructor encourages the patient to speak back the message, then 70% of the information is retained. By far the most effective retention, however, is by the patient demonstrating the skill back to the instructor.

> Hear it and I forget it
> Speak it and I remember
> Do it and I know. (ancient Chinese proverb)

The method for delivery of the message must also be considered. The aim is for the patient to identify the instructions with his or her own mouth (Fig 5-3). For this reason a traditional toothbrush demonstration on a plastic model is to be avoided. The patient sees a demonstration of a plastic model (with perfect teeth!) being brushed – *not* their own mouth. If the clinician orientates the model so that the lower arch is at the same orientation as the patient's lower arch then the patient has to crane their head to see it. If the clinician sits facing the patient and gains eye contact, the model is in reverse. Demonstration of the brushing of the maxillary teeth is especially difficult, as patients are not familiar with mirror images of the mouth.

The patient must be advised to bring his or her own toothbrush to the session (Fig 5-4). This is especially important if the patient uses a power brush, but they must be reminded to charge it! Alternatively, the practice may provide manual brushes of a suitable size for personal demonstration. A reminder on the reverse of the appointment card to bring in all oral cleaning devices will help. An option is to provide an individual starter pack to all new patients. It is a goodwill gesture, which will encourage the use of customised products. The patient is then able to try brushes or interdental tape with the clinician present, who can advise accordingly. Unfortunately, many of the hand

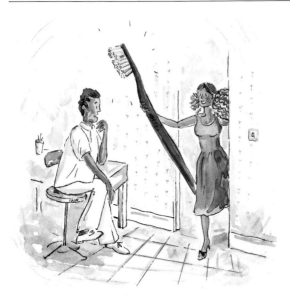

Fig 5-4 "I was thinking of something a little smaller!"

held interdental brushes are not available for sale in retail outlets and have to be ordered by mail order. This involves effort on the part of the patient and a possible time lag between order and supply, which can lead to a relapse in plaque control. If the practice is seriously promoting prevention of periodontal disease, then the brushes need to be available for patients to purchase on site. The various manufacturers do not standardise the colour of the handles according to the brush or wire diameter and this adds confusion to the choice. Communication is aided by recording in the records the precise interdental cleaning aid used, i.e. the brand name and the handle colour (Fig 5-5).

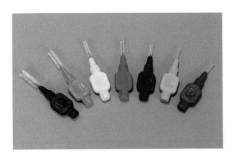

Fig 5-5 A range of short-handled colour-coded interdental brushes.

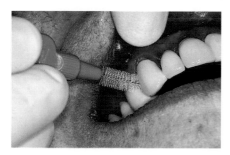

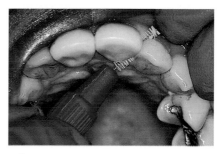

Fig 5-6 The interdental brushes must fit snugly between the teeth.

Fig 5-7 Approaching the interdental space from the palatal aspect.

Patients will only continue to buy products if they perceive them to be good value for money i.e. effective for the purpose of plaque removal and lasting for a "reasonable" period of time. Interdental brushes buckle and bend if they are too large for the interdental space, at which point the patient may become despondent and discontinue use. At every visit the brushes need to be checked for a snug fit (Fig 5-6).

As gingival recession occurs the interdental spaces become larger and the brushes need to be correspondingly larger to remove the plaque. Furcation sites will also become visible and cleansable with the correct brush, depending on the degree of furcation involvement.

Once manual dexterity has improved, the patient can be taught to approach the spaces from the lingual and palatal aspect as well as the buccal/labial approach (Fig 5-7). Patients may need to start with interdental brushes on a long handle, but again, as manual dexterity improves, a short-handled brush offers better control. Some examples of interdental cleaning aids available are detailed in Table 5-1. Examples of these aids in use are shown in Figs 5-8 to 5-10.

When should plaque control be carried out?
Whenever the patient has the time to commit to the regime in any 24-hour period. The advice "to socially clean" at other times is appropriate, but comprehensive plaque control must be conducted thoroughly at least once daily. The patient selects the specific period. Enforcement of a time when they have other commitments will lead to incomplete plaque removal and disease recurrence.

Table 5-1 **Interdental cleaning products.**

Product	Indication and requirements	Comments
Floss and tape	Tight interdental spaces with intact interdental papilla. good manual dexterity.	Useful in initial stages before recession.
Interdental brushes	Moderate-to-advanced bone loss with drifting and mobility, interdental spaces sufficiently large for the brush not to cause trauma to the hard and soft tissues, furcation spaces, prostheses on natural teeth and implants (e.g. bridge pontics).	Frequently damaged due to being forced into spaces. Handled brushes useful for the less dextrous patient. Good variety of sizes in short-handled models available for differing spaces.
Superfloss	Around fixed prostheses, good manual dexterity.	Possible to thread through spaces.
Flossettes	Limited use in tight contacts.	Limited use, less effective than interdental brushes.
Interspace brushes	Useful in instanding teeth, lone standing teeth, partially erupted teeth, and where a unit has been lost (e.g. denture abutment).	Easy to use.

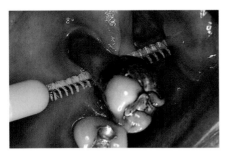

Fig 5-8 Furcation space cleaned by the interdental brush.

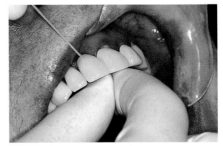

Fig 5-9 The use of superfloss to clean under a bridge pontic.

Continuation of the education process

To maintain patient compliance, education and motivation must be ongoing, requiring repetition at every visit, adaptation of the cleaning methods

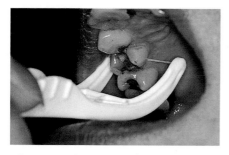

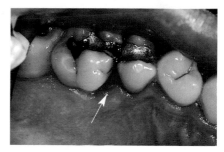

Fig 5-10 Flossettes (of limited use in tight contacts and less effective than interdental brushes).

Fig 5-11 Subtle inflammatory changes which may herald the onset of a lateral periodontal abscess.

and encouragement. Part of the education process is the demonstration of signs of disease and subtle soft tissue changes in the patient's mouth. Whilst charts and 3-D models are useful at the outset to explain the principles of the disease, the patient is more likely to relate to a personalised approach. Some patients are prone to recurrent periodontal abscesses (Fig 5-11). If they can be taught to recognise the tissue changes early before pain and inflammation are severe, they can seek advice sooner rather than later.

Patients should be taught to disclose plaque to see where the retention areas are, and if necessary to relate them to signs of inflammation. An active involvement in monitoring the plaque and bleeding scores with the dental hygienist will aid motivation. They can also be taught to smell the plaque retrieved from interdental areas on the interdental brushes and tape and therefore detect putrefaction (Fig 5-12). This can simply be related to the presence of mature microbial plaque that should have been removed more frequently!

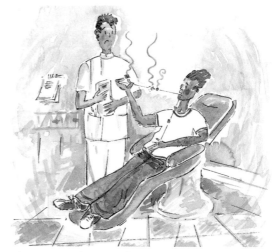

Fig 5-12 "I knew I should have cleaned out that curry last week."

Patients also need to be aware of the "difficult to reach" areas and taught how to access them. If the clinician finds an area difficult to instrument, then the patient will find that area difficult to maintain. It is worthwhile stopping to analyse how you, the clinician, overcome the problems and then explaining the solution to the patient. Examples include limited opening, overlaying of buccinator muscles onto posterior sites, a tight mentalis, or a strong gag reflex.

A motivated patient will be keen to try new techniques to save their teeth. The patient will also gradually learn that some areas of the mouth require more attention than others. This fact reinforces current clinical practice, i.e. certain areas of the mouth require more instrumentation and do not necessarily require polishing. In patients accustomed to a "regular six-monthly scale" selective polishing will need to be approached positively, otherwise patients may perceive that the clinician is "cutting corners!". Some long-term patients may find it difficult to convert from the hygienist undertaking scaling to talking about prevention. A suggestion is to stop and think, and discuss with the patient why the calculus reforms.

Reinforcement of the messages
Leaflets and posters reinforcing health messages are very valuable. The practitioner may encourage an interested dental nurse to qualify in oral health promotion, and utilise their skills within the practice. With desktop publishing, leaflets can be produced to promote practice protocols. Alternatively, toothbrush companies or the British Dental Health Foundation can supply them. Oral health promotion publications, videos and CD-ROMs may be purchased for the waiting room.

Time is very valuable in general practice and while it is important to have some social "chit chat" to place the patient at ease, some of the conversation time should be used to reinforce key health messages.

Smoking Cessation

All members of the team are in a prime position to educate patients about the detrimental effects of tobacco and the consequences of smoking. This position can be used to good advantage to give smoking cessation advice.

In 1998 the Department of Health published a white paper on tobacco use and highlighted the vital role members of the healthcare profession can play in smoking cessation. The department recommendations were that primary healthcare teams and hospitals should record the current smoking status of patients, and general practitioners should advise smokers to stop and record having done so at least once a year.

Any member of the dental team may give the appropriate advice, if they have received training. Tobacco use and strategies for smoking cessation are included in the curriculums of dental hygiene and dental therapy schools. Qualified hygienists and therapists are therefore suitably trained to advise patients on smoking cessation in a sensitive and informative manner.

The patient may have frequent appointments with the dental hygienist for the management of periodontitis. This offers opportunity for regular monitoring and reinforcement of smoking cessation. Dental hygienists are also good communicators and are therefore able to develop a rapport with their patients.

Time constraints are often quoted as a barrier to discussing smoking cessation with the patient. Evidence suggests that smoking is a major risk factor for periodontal diseases and, as a consequence, as important as plaque control in the disease stabilisation process (see Chapple and Gilbert 2002).

A team approach to smoking cessation
- Tackle smoking cessation advice as a team.
- Ensure collaboration and commitment from the whole team.
- Identify who should/could do what.
- Name who will have the active/support role.
- Share out the tasks amongst the team.

A practice meeting would be an opportunity to involve the entire team in advising patients in smoking cessation. A co-ordinator could consolidate the approach by arranging training and providing literature. Once established, it need only take a short time at each appointment for the clinician to reinforce the message and offer further advice.

Helping smokers to stop
The Health Education Authority in 1999 published guidance for the dental team to help smokers to quit. The recommendations were based on the "Four As" approach (Box 5-1).

Box 5-1

The "Four As" Approach

Ask *about smoking at every appointment. The clinician is to ask about smoking at every opportunity, to take a smoking history, and to record the information in the patient's clinical notes*

Advise *all smokers of the risk and to stop*

Assist *smokers to stop*

Arrange *a follow-up*

Taking a smoking history

If a current smoker:
- Why do they smoke?
- How many cigarettes do they smoke?
- How long have they been smoking?
- When do they smoke?
- Have they ever tried to stop?
- What happened when they tried to stop?
- Are they interested in stopping now or trying again?

If an ex-smoker:
- Make a note in their records.
- Remember to review periodically.

A tobacco assessment form is useful to determine the number of cigarettes smoked and the reasons for wanting to stop (Fig 5-13). People succeed in stopping smoking when they:
- are ready to stop
- understand their smoking patterns and their reasons for smoking
- know why they want to stop smoking now
- are prepared for how they will feel when they stop
- have developed alternative behaviours to replace their smoking habit
- make "staying stopped" a priority.

Date	
Name	
Address	

How many cigarettes do you smoke?	
How long have you been smoking this amount?	
Is the person most important to you a smoker?	YES / NO
Have you ever tried to stop smoking?	YES / NO
If yes, how many times?	
If yes, for how long have you stopped smoking?	
Are any of the following the main reasons for wanting to stop now?	
Your health	YES / NO
The expense	YES / NO
You don't like being addicted	YES / NO
Some other reason	YES / NO
If yes, please specify	

What will be your biggest problem in stopping smoking?

Fig 5-13 Tobacco use assessment form.

Advise

During the advice stage, it is appropriate to discuss the options of nicotine replacement therapies (Table 5-2) and provide written information. Raw *et al.* (1998) demonstrated that nicotine replacement doubled the rate of cessation. Smith *et al.* (1998) in an interventional study, using counselling by dentists and nicotine replacement therapy, obtained an 11% cessation rate after nine months. Very few people become addicted to the replacement (Silagy *et al.* 1996). However, replacement therapy is not recommended during pregnancy, for children under 16 years of age or for patients with heart problems. There are a range of products to suit the needs of the individual and their pat-

Table 5-2 **Nicotine replacement therapies.**

Product	Dosage	Recommendation
Nicotine skin patch★	5 mg / 16 hour release 10mg/ 16 hours 15mg/ 16 hours	Place on non-hairy skin and rotate site of patch. Commence with 15 mg and reduce to 5 mg
Nicotine gum★ (sugar free)	2 mg < 20 cigarettes a day 4 mg > 20 cigarettes a day	Chewed slowly for 30 minutes; heavy smokers use 4 mg gum
Nicotine nasal spray★	500 micrograms in a metered spray via nasal mucosa; maximum 64 sprays daily	For severe cravings on withdrawal when other aids are used; faster absorption than patch, gum or inhaler. May irritate nose
Nicotine inhaler★	10 mg cartridge between 6-12 cartridge daily, absorbed via oral mucosa	Nicotine cartridges fit inside a plastic mouthpiece; for smokers who need physical stimulus
Nicotine tablets (Microtab®)★	2 mg each hour for < 20 cigarettes day. 4 mg each hour for > 20 cigarettes a day.	Place under the tongue and allow to dissolve slowly
Amfebutamone/ Buproprion (Zyban® ‡)	150 mg tablets daily for 3 days, then reducing to 150 mg twice daily, maximum treatment 7–9 weeks.	Consult with medical practitioner; not recommended for patients under 18 years of age; contraindicated for: pregnancy, a history of epilepsy, eating disorders and bipolar disorder; side effect: xerostomia

★ Nicorette® products, Pharmacia Limited

‡ GlaxoSmithKline, Glaxo Wellcome UK Limited

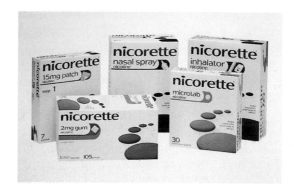

Fig 5-14 A range of smoking cessation products.

tern of addiction (Fig 5-14). The products are generally not available on the National Health Service. The replacement product should be continued for 10–12 weeks with gradual withdrawal over this period. If abstinence has not been achieved within 3 months, then treatment needs to be reviewed.

Assessing the patient's addiction using questionnaires such as the Fagerstrom Questionnaire (Table 5-3, Fig 5-15), helps to match the most appropriate replacement therapy to suit the needs of the individual.

How soon after waking do you smoke your first cigarette?	Within 5 mins	3
	6 – 30 mins	2
	3 – 60 mins	1
	after 60 mins	0
Do you find it difficult to refrain from smoking in places where it is forbidden?	Yes	1
	No	0
Which cigarette would you most hate to give up?	First in the morning	1
	All others	0
How many do you smoke a day?	31 or more	3
	21 to 30	2
	11 to 20	1
	10 or less	0
Do you smoke more frequently during the first hours after waking than during the rest of the day?	Yes	1
	No	0
Do you smoke when you are so ill that you spend most of the day in bed?	Yes	1
	No	0
	Total	

Fig 5-15 Assessing the patient's addiction – Fagerstrom questionnaire.

Table 5-3 **Interpretation of the Fagerstrom score.**

Points	Dependence	Recommended products
1–3	Low	2 mg gum, or Microtab®, or inhaler and will power.
4–5	Medium	Skin patch for regular smoking throughout the day; 2 mg gum or Microtab® for less regular smoking pattern; inhaler for craving of hand-to-mouth action.
6–7	High	Skin patch for regular smoking throughout the day or 4 mg gum or 4 mg Microtab®.
8–10	Very high	Nasal spray or 4 mg gum or 4 mg Microtab®.

Key points to cover with the smoker (Fig 5-16)
- Setting a date to stop.
- Reviewing past attempts – what helped or what hindered.
- Getting support of family and friends.
- Identifying potential problems and planning how to deal with them.

It is important to arrange a follow-up appointment. Cessation rates are more than doubled when follow-up contact is made with interested patients. Ideally, follow-up should be one to two weeks after the patient's chosen cessation date. If the patient is successful in stopping smoking, congratulate them and encourage them to remain smoke free. If unsuccessful, find the reason why and discuss how these problems might be overcome. Ask for a recommitment and review the patient's smoking status periodically. Most smokers make several attempts to stop before finally succeeding, so relapse is a normal part of the process.

Smoking Diary
A smoking diary (Fig 5-17) helps the patient to focus on the habit and to identify when and why they smoke. It is designed to provoke reflection on their automatic habits, routines, feelings and problems. A smoking diary is kept for two days, one day being at the weekend.

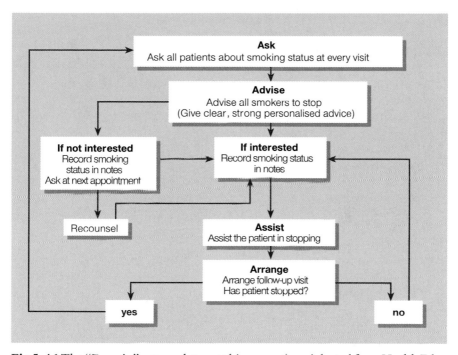

Fig 5-16 The "Four As" approach to smoking cessation. Adapted from Health Education Authority, Helping Smokers to Stop.

Time	What were you doing?	Who were you with?	How were you feeling?	How much did you enjoy it?	How much did you need it?

Fig 5-17 Smoking diary.

Assist

At the assist stage, the clinician can give practical advice, alleviate worries and answer questions. During this phase:

- Review the smoking diary.
- Advise on the benefits of stopping smoking.
- Emphasise health benefits.
- Stress the economic benefits.
- Promote the social acceptance.
- Reinforce the sense of self-control.
- Highlight well-being and quality of life.
- Encourage all practice staff to reinforce and support the patient's attempt to stop smoking.
- Provide information leaflets (ensure these are kept up to date).

Information
- National No Smoking Day.
- Quitline 0800 00 22 00.
- Quit website www.quit.org.uk.

Staying stopped
It is expected that the patient will feel cravings for a cigarette after stopping smoking. Help and supportive advice is essential during this period. Suggestions to ward off temptations are very useful and may include engaging in an alternative activity, such as exercise or chewing gum. Brushing the teeth is also helpful!

Withdrawal symptoms may include an increase in coughing, bowel upsets, dizziness, sleep disturbances, mood swings and hunger. These symptoms will subside over 2–3 weeks, hence support in the early days of cessation is invaluable.

The Health Education Authority recommended the "Four Ds" :
1. Delay the urge to smoke.
2. Deep breathe.
3. Drink water.
4. Do something else.

Key Points of Clinical Relevance

Effective patient education for the prevention of periodontal disease may be evaluated by:

- Self-recognition of signs of disease.
- Understanding of difficult-to-clean areas.
- Understanding the necessity to undertake interdental cleaning daily.
- Understanding that support is available, but that it is their responsibility to maintain plaque control.

Consistent, long-term motivation may be evaluated by:

- A commitment to efficient, effective plaque control FOR LIFE.
- Regular attendance.
- Cessation of smoking.
- Smoking cessation counselling should be an integral part of periodontal therapy and prevention.

Further Reading

Chapple ILC, Gilbert AD. Understanding Periodontal Diseases: Assessment and Diagnostic Procedures in Practice. London: Quintessence, 2002.

Watt R, Robinson M. Helping Smokers to Stop. A Guide for the Dental Team. London: Health Education Authority, 1999.

West R, McNeill A, Raw M. Smoking Cessation Guidelines for Health Professionals. Thorax 2000;55:987–999.

Raw M, McNeill A, West R. Smoking cessation guidelines for health professionals. A guide to effective smoking cessation, interventions for the health care system. Thorax 1998;53:Suppl 5:11–19.

Silagy C, Mant D, Fowler G, Lancaster T. Nicotine Replacement Therapy for Smoking Cessation (Cochrane Review). Oxford: Cochrane Library,1996.

Smith SE, Warnakulasuriya KA, Feyerabend C, Belcher M, Cooper DJ, Johnson NW. A smoking cessation programme conducted through dental practices in the UK. Br Dent J 1998;185: 299–303.

Chapter 6

Prevention of Oral Disease II: Diseases of the Hard Tissues

Aim

The aim of this chapter is to guide the dental team through the prevention of hard tissue tooth loss.

Outcome

The team members should have an understanding of the delivery of health messages to prevent dental caries, tooth erosion and abrasion.

Introduction

Dental hygienists and dental therapists have a role in educating the patient in the prevention of hard tissue tooth loss by dental caries, erosion and abrasion.

Dental Caries

Dental caries is a process of demineralisation caused by bacterial metabolism of fermentable carbohydrates. It is estimated that calcium hydroxyapatite will begin to dissolve when pH falls below 5.5. Dietary advice to prevent caries is therefore intended to reduce the duration and frequency of occasions when the pH of microbial plaque falls below the critical level.

In patients presenting for the management of periodontal disease, the emphasis is on prevention of secondary caries and primary root caries. This is because patients with a diagnosis of chronic periodontitis tend to be middle aged at the time of diagnosis and are more likely to present with previously restored dentitions. They may have lost teeth through either periodontal disease or caries and may wear partial dentures. They may have a medical or medication history which predisposes them to xerostomia and have recession of the periodontal tissues, exposing radicular dentine to demineralisation in the interproximal, buccal, lingual and furcation areas. Prevention is therefore aimed at identifying local risk factors, dietary factors and relevant habits.

Identifying plaque and local risk factors
One of the most effective methods is disclosing the plaque and demonstrating to the patient the plaque retained in a specific area. Disclosing the fitting surface of dentures is also useful.

Education subsequently involves selection of the most appropriate cleaning aid specifically to remove the plaque, bearing in mind the patient's manual dexterity and the availability of the product to be purchased.

Identifying dietary factors and habits
Dietary analysis may be done in two ways:
1. *24-hour analysis* – the patient documents everything eaten and drunk in the previous 24 hours.
2. *3-day analysis* – the patient documents everything eaten and drunk over a 3-day period. One day, at least, should be during the weekend.

Honesty is the key to success! (Fig 6-1).

The dental hygienist or therapist is then able to analyse the diet by circling in red every occasion when sugar is consumed. The education process can then commence with emphasis on reducing the frequency of non-milk extrinsic sugars and the suggestion of suitable alternatives.

The education process should involve discussion with the patient on the prevention of the loss of "key teeth" through understanding their oral cavity

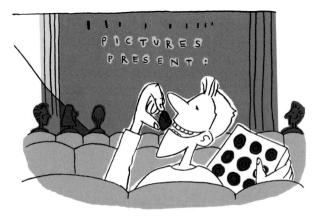

Fig 6-1 "I've only left out the bag of toffees I ate at the cinema!"

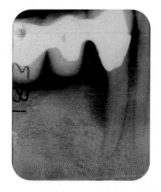
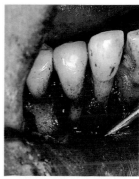

Fig 6-2 a and b Retention of key teeth, e.g. bridge abutments.

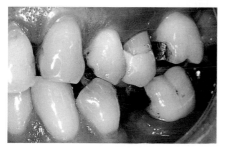
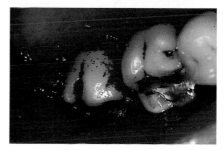

Fig 6-3 a and b A non-functional tooth and plaque accumulation from the palatal aspect.

and how it functions as a masticatory unit. The greater the understanding the more likely the personal commitment to preservation. Examples include education regarding abutment teeth for dentures and bridges and the consequences of extraction. A simple explanation of how loss of a bridge abutment may lead to denture provision will help the patient to focus on prevention (Fig 6-2). Education of the patient should focus on the maintenance of occlusal contacts to avoid non-functional teeth and subsequent plaque retention (Fig 6-3) and reinforcement of the importance of regular recall appointments for the early detection of interproximal and furcation caries.

Root caries can progress rapidly, and because the pulp may become involved at a relatively early stage, the consequences of late detection are substantial. Freshly exposed root surfaces will demineralise at a faster rate than sound enamel fissures in the same patient. This is because the root surfaces have not been exposed to calcium and phosphate ions in saliva, thus favouring demineralisation of the surface of the lesion, and because root dentine has a lower mineral content than enamel.

Patients who have chronic periodontitis complain of dentine hypersensitivity so frequently that the recommendation of a suitable desensitising dentifrice can be an automatic response. It is the dentist's responsibility to diagnose the problem as it is not within the hygienist's or therapist's remit. It is disappointing to lose a tooth through caries when the periodontal condition is stable after months of effort by all concerned!

Application of preventive agents

The hygienist or therapist may apply either fluoride gel to limit the demineralisation of calcified tissues or apply chlorhexidine gel as a varnish to temporarily reduce the cariogenic plaque load in a vulnerable area. Patients can be taught to apply the latter at home, either with a cotton bud or with an interdental brush.

Dental Erosion

All clinicians have a role in the recognition, recording and management of dental erosion. The tooth substance becomes demineralised and subsequently lost, but unlike caries, the process is not dependent upon bacterial metabolism. Erosive lesions tend to occur in plaque-free sites and in particular where gingival recession has occurred (Fig 6-4). Destruction of radicular dentine at sites exposed by migration of the periodontal tissues can be rapid. The patient in the maintenance phase of periodontal therapy may be particularly vulnerable to this form of tooth tissue loss. The acid source may be intrinsic or extrinsic.

Intrinsic sources in the middle-aged or elderly patient tend to be due to gastro-oesophageal reflux. Evidence may be seen on the palatal surfaces of the

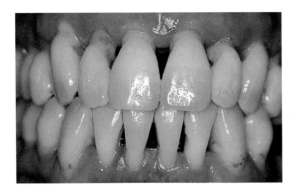

Fig 6-4 Erosion following gingival recession.

upper teeth, and the occlusal and buccal aspects of lower teeth. Mineralised tissue may be lost adjacent to the margins of restorations.

Extrinsic sources are acidic foods and drinks. These can lead to demineralisation of the labial and palatal surfaces of the upper anterior teeth. The extent and diversity of the tooth loss can be measured by an index such as the Smith and Knight's Index (1984). The hygienist or therapist can record the base line findings and take impressions for study models. These will be useful for educational, motivational and monitoring purposes.

Stages in management of dental erosion

Recognise and establish the aetiology. A careful medical, social and personal history may reveal the source of the acid. The questioning needs to be sensitive, especially if an eating disorder is suspected. A three-day dietary sheet is helpful.

The clinician should carefully identify causative factors and offer dietary counselling advice tailored to the needs of the individual. Frequently, compromises have to be reached between eating a healthy diet, including the recommended intake of fruit, and the exacerbation of erosion!

Advise the patient to avoid tooth brushing after a meal with an acidic component such as a glass of red wine, or after acid reflux. A bicarbonate of soda mouth rinse or a drink of milk will help neutralise the acid within saliva. The patient should confine acidic drinks to meal times and particularly avoid them before retiring to bed.

The clinician may apply fluoride topically to aid surface remineralisation or recommend fluoride rinses. Daily rinsing is more effective than a weekly regime, but requires greater compliance. Fluoride gels are available for home use but should be applied at a time separate from tooth cleaning. A Duraphat® dentifrice with a higher fluoride content of 2,800 ppm is also available (Table 6-1). The dentist and dental hygienist/therapist must work together in the prevention and management of dental erosion. Where the lesions have exposed dentine a desensitising dentifrice may be recommended or the dentist may advise restoration of eroded surfaces. Reinforcement of co-ordinated advice by the team will consolidate the health messages. Referral for the management of gastro-oesophageal reflux may be indicated.

Table 6-1 **Topical fluoride use.**

Product	Fluoride concentration	Usage	Application
Varnish	2.26%	Surgery	Twice a year
Acidulated phosphate fluoride gels	1.23%	Surgery	2–4 times a year
Gels	0.4%	Home	Daily
Rinses	0.05 %	Home	Daily
	0.2%	Home	Weekly
Dentifrice	2,800 ppm	Home	Daily

Dental Abrasion

This form of pathological tooth wear is detected by horizontal grooving of the enamel, cementum or dentine in the cervical region, usually of the buccal surfaces of the teeth.

The most common cause is overzealous tooth brushing in a horizontal plane. It may occur in patients with active periodontal disease because they are practising the horizontal scrub brushing technique rather than gingival sulcular cleaning such as the modified Bass technique (Fig 6-5). Toothbrushes that are worn out hold more paste which leads to potentially greater abrasion. A pea-sized amount of paste should be placed on a dry compact headed brush.

Patients in the maintenance phase are prone to abrasion lesions because the brushing technique has not been adapted to the new contours of the stable periodontium. Patients require instruction in the placement of the brush further apically to avoid grooving of the radicular dentine. This is equally important for the removal of supragingival plaque, which will accumulate if the brushing technique is ineffective.

The dentist and hygienist/therapist will need to be aware of other causes of abrasion such as ill-fitting dentures. Apparently, idiopathic causes of abrasion may be revealed and subsequently rectified by taking a detailed social history and noting habits such as cutting threads with the teeth and pipe smoking (Fig 6-6).

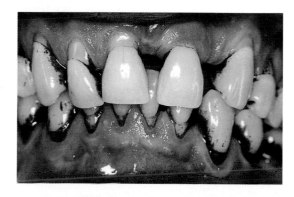

Fig 6-5 Abrasion due to an incorrect brushing technique.

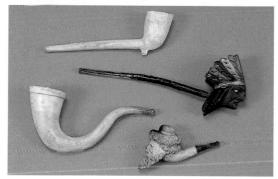

Fig 6-6 A collection of antique pipes.

Conclusion

Loss of tooth substance is of multifactorial aetiology. It is often not possible to attribute its cause to one factor. Gingival recession exposes the root surface to dental caries, erosion and abrasion. Educating the patient about the potential vulnerability of the root surfaces with simple messages is the most effective form of prevention.

Further Reading

Dietary Sugars and Human Disease. Committee on Medical Aspects of Food Policy. London: HMSO, 1989.

Smith BGN, Knight JK. An index for measuring the wear of teeth. Br Dent J 1984;156:435–438.

Chapter 7
Management of Periodontal Diseases

Aim

This chapter aims to consider the current classification of periodontal diseases; review best practice for screening and diagnosis of periodontal diseases; and give an overview of the periodontal therapy falling within the remit of a competent GDP.

Outcome

Having read this chapter the reader will be familiar with the screening, diagnosis and initial management of periodontal diseases in a general dental practice environment and be able to identify patients who would benefit from referral to a specialist.

The Role of the General Dental Practitioner

The GDP is the major provider of primary dental care and has a significant role in oral health education, screening to detect periodontal disease and following diagnosis to arrange appropriate care.

The dentist can coordinate and encourage a preventive approach to dental health throughout the practice, in the recognition that all members of the dental team can influence a patient's periodontal health. For example, every member of staff can and should encourage and support patients in smoking cessation. Dental nurses with an Oral Health Educator Certificate can manage Preventive Dental Units and assist individual patients to develop and maintain good oral hygiene. The success and stability of almost every aspect of dental care is dependent upon establishing a high standard of plaque control.

The dental hygienist has additional skills appropriate to the provision of an effective non-surgical course of periodontal therapy. The majority of periodontal disease is of a chronic form and only 8% of dentate adults in the UK have loss of attachment of 6 mm or more. Thus, the number of patients requiring complex specialist treatment is low and the delegation of initial non-surgical periodontal care to a dental hygienist is appropriate due to the high quality and reduced cost of treatment. The role of the hygienist in long-term maintenance of periodontal health has been well documented. Studies of the long-term outcome of periodontal treatment have demonstrated convincingly that maintenance of a high standard of oral hygiene prevents or at least reduces the progression of periodontal diseases.

In the provision of restorative dental care (Chapter 10) the dentist should work closely with the dental technician to ensure that both fixed and removable prostheses are designed and constructed to facilitate oral hygiene and avoid occlusal trauma to the remaining teeth (Chapter 9). Thus, there are relatively few periodontal patients who cannot be treated and maintained to high standards within the confines of a general dental practice and the whole dental team has a role to play in the prevention of periodontal disease.

Periodontal disease in its early stages causes few, if any, symptoms and patients are often unaware that they have a problem. It is therefore the duty of the GDP to monitor and screen patients for the presence of periodontal diseases. Where clinical findings indicate disease, relevant radiographs should be obtained. The practitioner should, following diagnosis, develop a treatment plan with specified therapeutic outcomes.

The long-term outcome of periodontal therapy is dependent upon patient compliance. It should be recognised that not all patients will be psychologically or physically capable of complying with the optimal standard of oral hygiene and some may even decline therapy. Nevertheless, all patients have the right to make an informed choice in relation to periodontal management.

All periodontal assessments should be recorded in the clinical notes. In particular probing pocket depths, clinical attachment levels, bleeding sites, plaque scores and mobility should be recorded. All clinically successful modalities of periodontal therapy include the substantial reduction of subgingival plaque. The outcome of periodontal therapy should be assessed in relation to patient comfort and aesthetics. Once periodontal stability has been achieved it is essential to arrange a supportive care programme.

Clinical Guidelines for Screening

Periodontal diseases can occur in any patient regardless of age. It is therefore vital to perform a periodontal screening examination for all patients at reg-

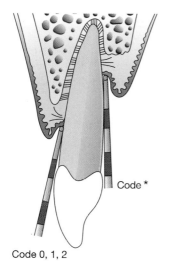

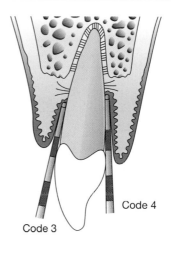

Fig 7-1a Line diagram illustrating the BPE coding system 0, 1, 2 ı *.

Fig 7-1b Diagram illustrating the BPE coding system for codes 3 and 4.

ular intervals. An assessment of each individual patient's "risk" of developing periodontal disease will influence the frequency of maintenance. The British Society of Periodontology and the Faculty of General Dental Practitioners of the Royal College of Surgeons of England have both produced clinical guidelines recommending routine screening for periodontal disease.

The Basic Periodontal Examination (BPE) is the recommended screening method. The use of BPE is an essential feature in orthodontic and complex restorative treatment planning. The benefits and limitations of the BPE are detailed in the first book of the Quintessentials series (Chapple and Gilbert 2002). The BPE codes and their relevance to periodontal treatment needs are shown in Table 7-1 and Fig 7-1.

Table 7-2 summarises the recommendations for radiographic examination of patients when clinical examination reveals the presence of periodontal disease. A variety of panoramic radiographic equipment is available. Panoramic films are of use only when good quality imaging of the anterior sextants can be achieved.

Table 7-1 **The Basic Periodontal Examination (BPE) codes.**

BPE Code		Clinical status	Treatment needs
0	Coloured band is completely visible no calculus no gingival bleeding	Healthy periodontium	Repeat screening.
1	Coloured band is completely visible no calculus plaque and gingival bleeding	Gingivitis	Oral hygiene instruction.
2	Calculus supra- and or subgingival, iatrogenic plaque retention factors (prfs), no pockets >3 mm coloured band completely visible	Gingivitis	Oral hygiene instruction, scaling, remove plaque retention factors.
3	Coloured area of the probe remains partly visible in the deepest pocket in the sextant	Periodontitis, shallow pocketing 5 mm or less	Non-surgical periodontal care within remit of general dental practitioner.
4	Coloured area of probe completely disappears	Periodontitis, deep pockets ≥ 5.5 mm	May require complex specialist periodontal care.
★	Annotates other codes	Furcation involvement or attachment loss exceeding 7 mm in total	Signifies poor prognosis. Consider specialist opinion.

Diagnosis

Screening using the BPE can highlight the presence of periodontal disease, but a detailed history and examination are required to reach a diagnosis and formulate a detailed treatment plan. These topics are detailed in Chapple and Gilbert 2002. A periodontal examination should include:

Table 7-2 **Selection criteria for radiographic examination in patients with periodontal disease.**

Disease	Distribution	Severity	Radiograph
Gingivitis			None
Periodontitis	generalised	mild (LOA ≤ 3mm)	DPT
		moderate (LOA >3mm but <5mm)	DPT and supplemental films of localised areas (e.g. furcation involvements) using PAs or vertical bitewings
		severe (LOA >5mm)	periapicals of standing teeth or DPT if considering clearance
Periodontitis	localised – posterior teeth only affected	mild	horizontal bitewings
		moderate	vertical bitewings
		severe	periapicals of affected teeth or DPT initially ± supplemental PAs
Periodontitis	localised – anterior teeth only affected	mild	periapicals of affected teeth or DPT initially ± supplemental PAs
		moderate	as above
		severe	as above
Periodontitis	localised involving anterior and posterior teeth	mild	DPT
		moderate	DPT initially ± vertical bitewings for posteriors ± PAs for anterior teeth
		severe	periapicals of standing teeth or DPT initially ± supplemental PAs

LOA = loss of attachment; DPT = dental pantomograph; PA = periapical x-ray

- Standard of oral hygiene, location and quantity of plaque and calculus deposits.
- Note of plaque retention factors.
- Assessment of the gingiva for signs of inflammation, recession and hyperplasia.
- Periodontal probing, recording probing pocket depths, bleeding on probing and suppuration.
- Location of furcation defects.
- Presence and degree of tooth mobility.
- Occlusal assessment to include static and dynamic function, wear faceting and premature contacts.
- Oral mucosal assessment for signs of systemic diseases.
- Radiographic examination (see Table 7-2).

Classification of periodontal diseases

The classification of periodontal diseases is complex. In addition to thorough clinical examination, a detailed social, medical and family history should be obtained to assist diagnosis. The most recent classification resulting from the 1999 Illinois International Workshop for the Classification of Periodontal Diseases and Conditions is summarised in Table 7-3. A detailed appraisal of this system is discussed in Chapple and Gilbert 2002.

This classification attempts to relate disease to differing aetiologies, prognosis and treatment modalities. The difference between chronic (Fig 7-2) and aggressive (Fig 7-3) forms of periodontitis are summarised in Table 7-4 and Table 7-5 gives details of the differences between periodontal and periapical abscesses. It is important to note that there is no indication to use systemic antimicrobial drugs in the management of chronic periodontitis, but they do have a role in the management of aggressive disease. It is not the remit of this book to discuss the clinical management of the most common periodontal diseases; this will be covered in the third book of the present series, *Successful Periodontal Therapy: A Non-Surgical Approach*.

Table 7-3 **Classifications of gingival and periodontal diseases (International Workshop 1999).**

Gingival diseases

Dental plaque-induced gingival diseases	Gingivitis associated with dental plaque only Gingival diseases modified by systemic factors Gingival diseases modified by medications Gingival diseases modified by malnutrition
Non-plaque-induced gingival lesions	Gingival diseases of specific bacterial origin Gingival diseases of viral origin Gingival diseases of fungal origin Gingival lesions of genetic origin Gingival manifestations of systemic conditions Traumatic lesions Foreign body reactions Not otherwise specified (NOS)

Periodontal diseases

Chronic periodontitis	Localised Generalised
Aggressive periodontitis	Localised Generalised
Necrotising periodontal diseases	Necrotising ulcerative gingivitis Necrotising ulcerative periodontitis Abscesses of the periodontium
Periodontitis associated with endodontic lesions	
Developmental or acquired deformities and conditions	
Periodontitis as a manifestation of systemic diseases	Haematological disorders Genetic disorders Not otherwise specified (NOS)

Table 7-4 **Comparison of the main features of chronic and aggressive periodontitis.**

	Aggressive periodontitis (Fig 7-3)	Chronic periodontitis (Fig 7-2)
Male:female ratio	Equal incidence in males and females	Increased incidence in males
Incidence	Rare (less than 5% of population at risk)	Common (54% of population with ≥ 4 mm attachment loss)
Age of onset	Forms occur in mixed dentition, at puberty and early adulthood	May commence in teenagers but usually diagnosis is after 30 years of age
Rate of progression	Rapid rate of tissue destruction	Average slow progression with "random burst" pattern
Microbiology	Specific periodontal pathogens include *actinobacillus actinomycetemcomitans, porphyromonas gingivalis, fusobacterium nucleatum* and spirochaetes	Mixed non-specific flora, increased proportion gram-negative organisms; some organisms specifically linked: *porphyromonas gingivalis, tanerella forsythensis, treponema denticola*
Host defence	Hypo- and hyper-responsive inflammatory phenotypes have been reported	Hyper-inflammatory/ immune response which can contribute to tissue destruction
Oral hygiene	Good oral hygiene	Disease correlates with worsening oral hygiene
Management	May benefit from adjunctive systemic antimicrobials	Responds well to simple removal of microbial deposits; no indication for the use of systemic antimicrobials

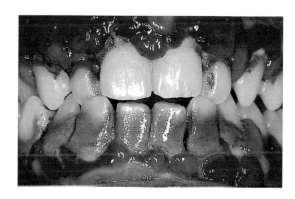

Fig 7-2 Chronic periodontitis associated with poor levels of oral hygiene.

Fig 7-3 a and b Radiographic and clinical features of aggressive periodontitis.

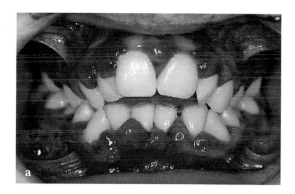

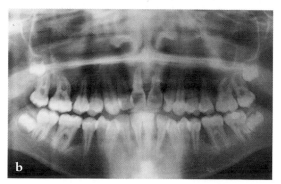

Table 7-5 **Differences between lateral periodontal and periapical abscess.**

	Lateral periodontal abscess	Periapical abscess
Vitality of tooth	Usually vital	Non-vital; beware, multi-rooted teeth may respond
Pain	Less severe than apical abscess	Very severe; disturbs sleep usually
Discharge	Through pocket	Usually over apex, may be at gingival margin
Swelling	On attached gingiva	Over apex
Area of maximum tenderness	On attached gingiva	Over apex
Timing	Usually swelling precedes pain	Usually pain before swelling
Tenderness to percussion	Usually not very; more on lateral movement	Extreme tenderness to apical pressure
Pocketing	Usually present	Not necessarily present
History of trauma or previous filling	Not necessarily	Usually
Previous symptoms of pulpitis	Not necessarily	Often
Appearance on radiograph	Marginal bone loss visible	May show apical radiolucency if present 10 days or more

Periodontal Treatment in the Primary Care Sector

The British Society of Periodontology has issued a policy document *Referral Policy and Parameters of Care* (2001) which outlines a referral policy guideline for patients with a diagnosis of periodontitis dependent upon the findings of a BPE screen. The decision to refer patients to either specialist practitioners or hospital consultants is dependent upon the:

- GDP's knowledge and ability to treat periodontal patients, which may vary considerably
- patient's motivation to seek a specialist opinion or treatment
- age and general health of the patient
- complexity of treatment required
- form of periodontitis diagnosed
- proximity of local specialist services.

In the 1998 Office for National Statistics Adult Dental Health Survey, 73% of dentate adults had some calculus and 54% periodontal pocketing of 4 mm or more. The prevalence of periodontal disease is such that most patients will need to be managed in a primary care setting. The general dental practitioner will need to be skilled in:

- The screening of patients, and selection of relevant radiographs.
- Reaching a diagnosis and formulating a treatment plan with defined therapeutic goals.
- The provision of non-surgical care (in conjunction with the dental hygienist).
- Monitoring the response to initial therapy.

The rate of progression of periodontal disease varies in each person. For each individual patient an assessment of the rate of disease progression must be made in relation to age and other associated risk factors, e.g. general health, smoking and oral hygiene practices. The patient should be given a clear explanation of their oral status in terms that they can understand. Dental radiographs, hand mirrors and probes can be used to demonstrate the presence of periodontal breakdown in the patient's mouth.

The consequences of failing to accept treatment must be made clear. It is important to remember that not every patient will be capable of, or motivated to, embark upon a course of periodontal treatment. Nevertheless, every patient should have treatment options explained so that they can exercise an informed choice and information given must be documented in their clinical records. For reasons of systemic disease or problems with plaque control or lack of motivation, appropriate treatment to control disease may be deferred or declined.

The treatment of periodontitis is fundamentally dependent upon the patient's motivation, manual dexterity and compliance. Thus the outcome of care may be difficult to predict. Indeed in some cases, because of severity and extent of disease, age or poor health of the patient, a treatment that will reduce but not control disease progression may be selected. In these cases, initial therapy to improve oral hygiene and remove supragingival calculus may be the end-point.

It is good clinical practice (and a recommendation of the dental defence organisations) that a written record of all periodontal assessments is kept. In particular, practitioners should record probing pocket depths, attachment levels, bleeding sites, plaque scores and mobility. Patient compliance and healing are variable and so it is essential to monitor their individual response to therapy and record findings. Remember that the objective of periodontal care is to provide an appropriate dentition to meet the individual patient's aesthetic and functional needs. The end-point of treatment has to be selected for each case.

Initial periodontal therapy, as provided in a primary care setting by general dental practitioners and dental hygienists, is effective provided that, once periodontal disease is controlled, a supportive care programme is arranged.

There are some patients in whom either the outcome of periodontal therapy is inexplicably poor or complex therapy is indicated. It is the GDP who can identify and select those patients who would benefit from referral for specialist care. A specialist opinion should be sought after completion of

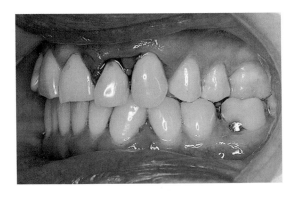

Fig 7-4 Despite good oral hygiene the deep periodontal pocket 22 shows bleeding after probing indicative of active periodontitis.

cause-related therapy in a practice setting. Where active periodontal pocketing persists after non-surgical periodontal therapy (Fig 7-4) in a patient with good oral hygiene, it is appropriate to refer for the provision of complex periodontal therapy such as periodontal surgery. Patients with inadequate oral hygiene and a diagnosis of chronic periodontitis should receive further non-surgical treatment and demonstrate sufficient motivation and manual dexterity to improve plaque control prior to warranting specialist referral. However, remember that all patients have a "right" to a second opinion through referral.

Selection criteria for specialist referral

The following groups of patients are at risk of severe periodontal disease or complications arising from therapy. Early referral for specialist opinion following detection of periodontal disease may be appropriate:

1. Patients with medical conditions predisposing to periodontal disease e.g. cyclic neutropenia, organ transplants with drug-induced overgrowth, poorly controlled diabetes, immunosupression and renal failure or transplant (Fig 7-5).
2. Patients at special risk of complications arising from dental treatment, e.g. those on anticoagulant therapy, those with prosthetic heart valves, previous rheumatic fever/infective endocarditis or significant heart murmur and immunosupression (Fig 7-6).
3. Patients with a diagnosis of aggressive periodontitis, e.g. localised aggressive periodontitis or generalised aggressive periodontitis (Fig 7-7).
4. Complex restorative treatment planning for periodontal cases, e.g. combined periodontal and endodontic lesions (Fig 7-8), combined periodontal and orthodontic treatment, planning of fixed prosthodontics and implants, and potential need for periodontal surgery.

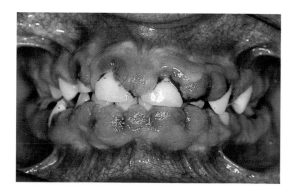

Fig 7-5 Gingival overgrowth attributed to ciclosporin in a renal transplant patient.

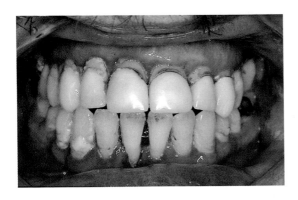

Fig 7-6 Active periodontitis in an HIV positive patient.

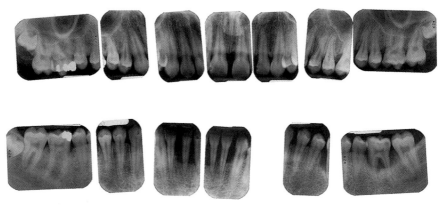

Fig 7-7 Typical radiographic features of aggressive periodontitis.

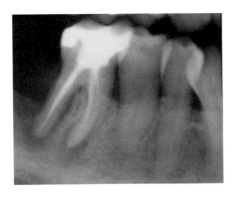

Fig 7-8 Radiograph showing a combined periodontal-endodontic lesion.

The Clinical Audit Committee of the Royal College of Surgeons of England, with help from the British Society of Periodontology, produced an index of treatment needs for periodontal treatment assessment. This codes complexity in a simplistic manner with the addition of a list of modifying factors that are relevant to periodontal treatment and an outline of medical histories that may significantly influence clinical management. It is in essence a complexity index, which does not take into consideration either aspects of patient motivation or criteria for prioritisation of treatment. The criteria used to select the complexity grade and relevant modifying factors are outlined in Table 7-6. The complexity index is a useful tool for providing guidance about the best environment for treatment to be performed, according to its complexity. One area of possible ambiguity is the management of smokers with a BPE of 4 in any sextant. Recent research has shown that the response

Table 7-6 **Complexities of periodontal treatment codes.**

Criteria	Complexity rating
Modifying factors	Modifying factors can only increase complexity by one increment. Multiple factors not cumulative
Medical history	Significant medical history increases complexity by one increment
BPE score 1-3 in any sextant	Complexity 1
BPE score 4 in any sextant; surgery involving periodontal tissues	Complexity 2
Surgery associated with osseointegrated implants; surgery involving periodontal tissue augmentation; BPE score 4 in any sextant, plus one or more of the following factors: patients under 35 years of age; smoking 10+ cigarettes per day; medical factor directly affecting periodontal tissues; adverse root morphology; rapid periodontal breakdown >2mm attachment loss in a year	Complexity 3

of smokers to non-surgical periodontal treatment is impaired and surgical treatment in particular will not produce a sustained clinical benefit. The recommended outcome of the complexity rating is:
- Complexity 1 cases may be treated in general practice.
- Complexity 2 cases can be either treated by the general practitioner or referred.
- Complexity 3 cases are mostly referred to a specialist periodontist.

It is not possible to be absolute in determining strict referral guidelines. Sometimes apparently simple periodontal treatment may need to be provided by specialists as an integral part of a more complex treatment plan. In other situations, local service demands and contracts may result in a referral being declined.

Non-surgical periodontal therapy

The objective of "cause-related therapy" is elimination and prevention of reformation of bacterial deposits on tooth and root surfaces. Periodontal disease affects specific sites to varying degrees and so it is essential to record in detail the location and severity of periodontal disease before commencing treatment. Examples of periodontal charting schemes are illustrated in Figs 3-7 to 3-10, and 7-9. Computer-generated charting systems are also available.

Healing after periodontal therapy may continue for up to six months. Charting after a suitable period for healing has elapsed (6–12 weeks minimum) permits an accurate assessment of a patient's response to therapy and long-term monitoring of the disease process. In addition, charts can be used for individual patient motivation and education. Cause-related or initial periodontal therapy comprises:
- Patient motivation.
- Oral health education.
- Removal of plaque retention factors.
- Supragingival scaling.
- Subgingival scaling.
- Root surface debridement.
- Occlusal equilibration.
- Chemical plaque control (for acute conditions).

The oral health education of a patient underpins effective motivation. Once the patient fully understands the role of bacterial plaque as the causative agent in caries and periodontal disease, subsequent oral hygiene instruction will have relevance. A dental health educator or dental hygienist can provide this phase of care.

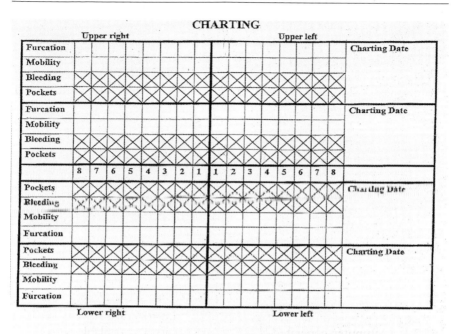

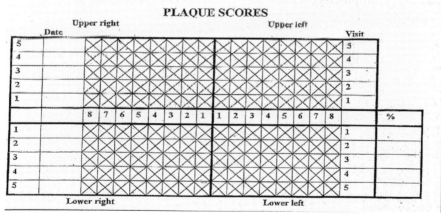

Fig 7-9 a Examples of charting systems available for recording periodontal indices.

FP25P

Surname .... Practice Ref. ....

First Forename .... Dentist's Name ....

Date of Birth ....

CPITN Score

on ....

Date of initial assessment ....

INITIAL																		
Mobility																		
Plaque	B																	
	P																	
Gingival Bleeding	B																	
	P																	
Pocket Depth	B																	
	P																	
Tooth Notation		**8**	**7**	**6**	**5**	**4**	**3**	**2**	**1**	**1**	**2**	**3**	**4**	**5**	**6**	**7**	**8**	
Pocket Depth	L																	
	B																	
Gingival Bleeding	L																	
	B																	
Plaque	L																	
	B																	
Mobility																		

UPPER

LOWER

Date of review assessment ....

REVIEW																		
Mobility																		
Plaque	B																	
	P																	
Gingival Bleeding	B																	
	P																	
Pocket Depth	B																	
	P																	
Tooth Notation		**8**	**7**	**6**	**5**	**4**	**3**	**2**	**1**	**1**	**2**	**3**	**4**	**5**	**6**	**7**	**8**	
Pocket Depth	L																	
	B																	
Gingival Bleeding	L																	
	B																	
Plaque	L																	
	B																	
Mobility																		

UPPER

LOWER

Gingival Recession

Overhanging margins at

Furcation involvement at

NATIONAL HEALTH SERVICE DENTAL RECORD - PERIODONTAL

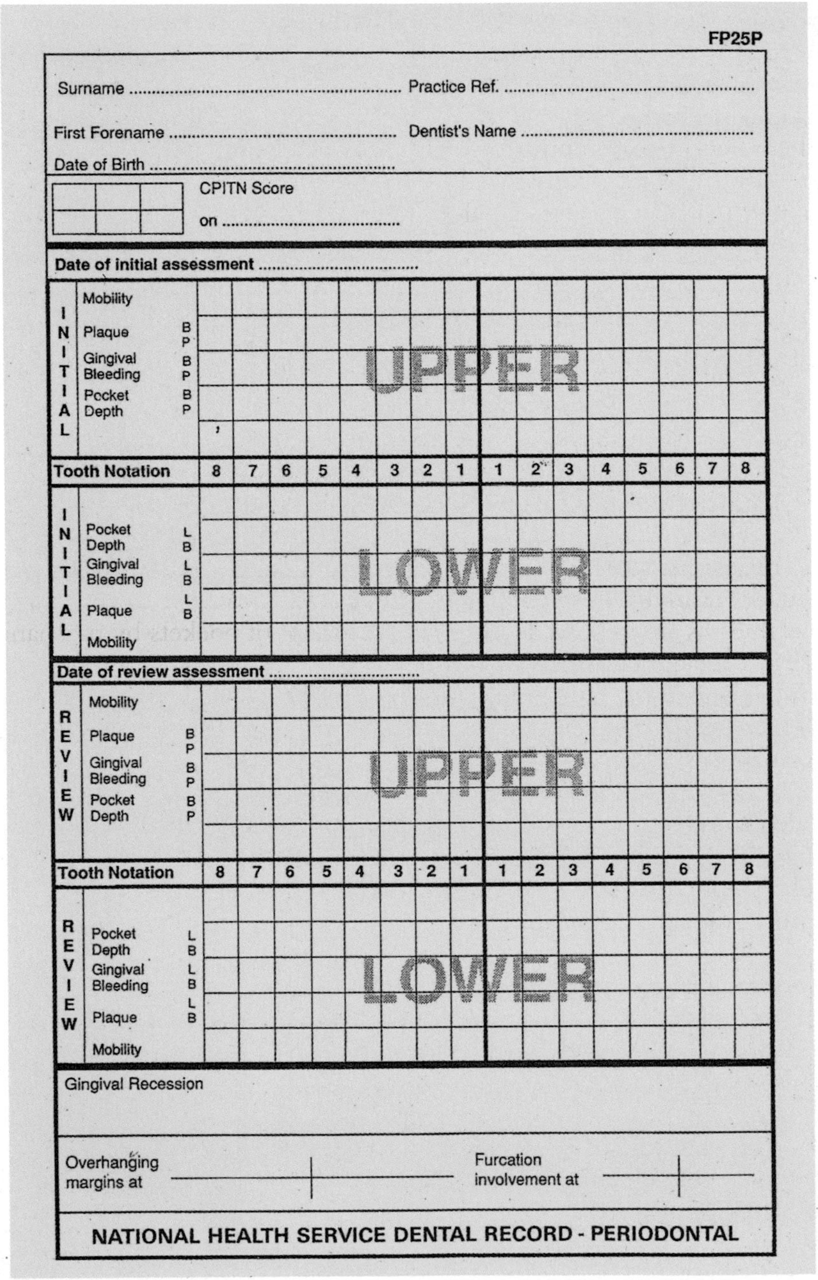

Fig 7-9 b Six probing pocket depth measures are needed per tooth.

Plaque retention factors may be natural (crowding, developmental grooves, enamel pearls, calculus) or iatrogenic (poor margins or overcontoured restorations as detailed in Chapter 10).

Either a dentifrice or mouth rinse may deliver chemical plaque control. The most effective agents contain chlorhexidine. Problems of altered taste sensation, staining and increased calculus formation may arise with chlorhexidine mouth rinse preparations. Triclosan presented in combination with a polymer designed to increase substantivity or zinc also provides effective antiplaque activity for the control of gingivitis but is ineffective in the management of periodontal pocketing. An account of occlusal therapy in relation to periodontal diseases is presented in Chapter 9.

Historically, subgingival instrumentation has been performed with the objective of total removal of subgingival deposits, leaving a smooth root surface. It has been shown that this is rarely achieved and yet periodontal therapy is effective. Recent studies have shown that 90% of the lipopolysaccharide (LPS or endotoxin) associated with periodontally involved root surfaces is found within the loosely adherent plaque layer and can be easily removed. Several terms are used to describe the treatment of pockets by mechanical therapy. These include:
- *Subgingival scaling* – the removal of subgingival calculus.
- *Root planing* – the removal of subgingival plaque, calculus and necrotic cementum.
- *Root surface debridement (or instrumentation)* – the removal of calculus and adequate subgingival loosely adherent plaque to facilitate periodontal healing. Root surface debridement is a less aggressive procedure than root planing and aims to preserve as much cementum as possible, without compromising therapeutic outcomes.

Corrective Therapy
For a more detailed account of this topic please refer to the third book in the present series (*Successful Periodontal Therapy: A Non-Surgical Approach*). A patient demonstrating compliance with plaque control may be considered for corrective therapy. This may comprise:
- Further root surface debridement in residual active sites.
- Management of combined periodontal and endodontic lesions.
- Replacement of defective restorations.
- Provision of partial dentures.
- Placement and reconstruction of osseointegrated implants.
- Periodontal surgery.

Initial or cause-related therapy is usually performed before decisions regarding the use of periodontal surgery can be taken. Patients who achieve good standards of oral hygiene after thorough root surface debridement but have periodontal disease activity (increasing pocket depths and/or bleeding on probing) are potential candidates for periodontal surgery.

Periodontal surgery may be indicated where there is impaired access for scaling and root surface debridement. The ability to perform adequate root surface instrumentation is reduced:
- in deeper (>5 mm) periodontal pockets
- on wider tooth surfaces
- by the presence of root fissures
- by the presence of root concavities
- by furcations
- by the presence of faulty margins on subgingival restorations.

Surgery also has a role where access is impaired for self-performed plaque control. The morphology of the dentogingival area has a significant affect on even a well motivated and manually dexterous patient's ability to achieve plaque control, in particular in areas of extensive gingival overgrowth and fibrous retromolar or tuberosity tissue. High fraenal attachments and interdental craters can create significant plaque control problems. Periodontal surgery may therefore be used to:
- gain access for thorough scaling and root surface debridement
- establish a gingival morphology conducive to good plaque control at home
- reduce pocket depths either by tissue removal, formation of a long junctional epithelium or regeneration of new connective tissue attachment
- shift the gingival margin such that it lies apical to plaque retaining restorations
- increase clinical crown length to permit preparation of retentive indirect restorations with supragingival margins (crown lengthening).

There are contraindications to periodontal surgery. Case selection is of fundamental importance in achieving a long-term improvement in the periodontal health of the patient. Patient compliance is essential to ensure optimal postoperative care. A patient who is not able or motivated to cooperate during the initial phase of cause-related therapy should not proceed to surgery, since the outcome, even if showing short-term gain, will be compromised as periodontal breakdown inevitably recurs. Smoking is not only a major risk factor for periodontal disease progression but has also been shown to impair healing after both non-surgical and surgical therapy. In comparison to non-smokers, less pocket depth reduction and smaller improvements in clinical attachment gain are observed after surgical therapy in smokers. It has been estimated that tissue blood supply and healing may not recover for up to one year after smoking cessation is commenced.

There are few other absolute contraindications; however, care must be taken in planning surgery for medically compromised patients, e.g. for those with cardiovascular disease including hypertension, angina pectoris, myocardial infarct, anticoagulation treatment, risk of bacterial endocarditis and organ transplant patients in whom antihypertensive therapy is associated with gingival overgrowth.

Periodontal surgery may be classified as:

1. *Access surgery* – designed to provide visual and technical access for thorough debridement in deep sites.
2. *Resective surgery* – for removal of excess soft tissue in gingival overgrowth or apical relocation of gingival margins in the management of pocketing.
3. *Regenerative surgery* – although less predictable, this form of surgery is reported to regenerate the periodontal attachment complex, i.e. cementum, periodontal ligament and bone.
4. *Periodontal plastic surgery* – which aims to correct muco-gingival defects, e.g. clefts resulting from localised gingival recession via grafting or similar procedures (Fig 7-10).

Adjunctive antimicrobial therapy
For a more detailed account of this topic see the third book in the present series. Briefly:

There is no indication for the regular or routine use of systemic antibiotics in the management of chronic periodontal diseases. The Standing Medical

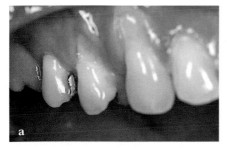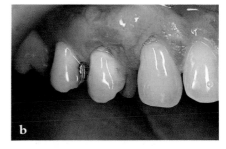

Fig 7-10 Gingival recession (a) pre- and (b) post-connective tissue grafting.

Advisory Committee of the Department of Health advocates caution in the use of antimicrobials by dental practitioners due to risk of increased drug resistance of bacteria throughout the population in general. The increase in methicillin-resistant *Staphylococcus aureus* (MRSA) can be attributed largely to overuse of antimicrobial drugs. Patients who smoke will benefit less from the adjunctive use of antibiotics. The efficacy of adjunctive antibiotics in periodontal therapy is dependent upon thorough mechanical debridement, which will by definition disrupt the biofilm structure of subgingival plaque.

There is evidence that systemic antibiotics (provided they are used as an adjunct to mechanical therapy) can enhance the clinical outcome for aggressive periodontitis. Aggressive periodontal disease, in which there is reported to be an increased prevalence of specific periodontal pathogens, responds to systemic antimicrobial therapy.

Oral sites including the tongue, fauces, floor of mouth and saliva will harbour periodontal pathogens; hence the need for a systemic drug to "cleanse" the whole oral environment and prevent re-colonisation of pockets with a pathogenic flora. Also, the tetracycline drugs will reduce collagenase production by the patient's polymorphonuclear leucocytes; hence reducing the potential for tissue destruction by an over-exuberant host response.

Topical antimicrobials are designed to produce high drug levels within the periodontal pocket. They are intended for use in local, non-responding sites where a diagnosis of chronic periodontitis has been made. The efficacy of such preparations is questionable. They should only be considered if patients are achieving an excellent standard of oral hygiene and the site has failed to heal despite repeated mechanical therapy. These are discussed in more detail in the third book in the present series.

Monitoring

Individual responses to periodontal therapy vary considerably and are difficult to predict. It is essential therefore to monitor both the patient's compliance with oral hygiene techniques and the tissue response to therapy. Compliance is best monitored using plaque and gingival indices, and observing calculus and stain reformation. Tissue response can be assessed using clinical attachment levels, probing pocket depths, bleeding on probing and the recording of recession. Comparison with pretreatment records will demonstrate the healing response.

At least six weeks should pass after root surface instrumentation before reassessment takes place. Indeed, improvements in clinical status may continue for up to six months after conventional non-surgical therapy. Any clinical improvement following either surgical or non-surgical periodontal therapy can only be sustained within a well-planned supportive care (maintenance) programme.

Key Points

- The GDP has a responsibility to screen and monitor patients for periodontal diseases.
- The minimum screening examination acceptable is a BPE (a clinical assessment with appropriate radiographic examination).
- A periodontal diagnosis should be made and documented in the notes.
- Where disease is detected a treatment plan should be instituted with clear therapeutic goals.
- Patients must always be fully informed of the diagnosis, treatment options and prognosis.
- It is essential to monitor the response to therapy.
- Always keep full records in the clinical notes, particularly taking care to record periodontal indices and advice given regarding oral hygiene and smoking cessation.
- Do not underestimate the need for long-term periodontal maintenance; patients must be educated to appreciate that they are making a life-long commitment when accepting periodontal treatment.

Further Reading

Adult Antimicrobial Prescribing in Primary Dental Care for General Dental Practitioners. Faculty of General Dental Practitioners (UK). London: The Royal College of Surgeons of England, 2000.

Adult Dental Health Survey. London: Office for National Statistics, 1998.

Ahrens G, Bulblitz KA. Parodontalerkrankungen und Behandlungsbedarf der Hamburger Bevölkerung Eine epidemiologische Studie an 11.305 Probanden. Dtsch Zahnärztl Z 1987;42:433–437.

Armitage GC. Development of a classification system for periodontal diseases and conditions. Ann Periodontol 1999;4:1–7.

British Society of Periodontology. Periodontology in General Dental Practice in the United Kingdom. A Policy Statement. London: BSP, 2001.

British Society of Periodontology. Referral Policy and Parameters of Care. London: BSP, 2001.

Standing Medical Advisory Committee (SMAC). The Path of Least Resistance. London: Department of Health, 1998.

Chapter 8

Orthodontics and Periodontal Health

Aim

This chapter aims to consider the relationship between malocclusion and periodontal health and disease states and to identify the potential risks to periodontal health that orthodontic treatment may introduce.

Outcome

At the end of this chapter the practitioner should be able to identify patients in whom orthodontic treatment may be a risk to their periodontal health and be familiar with options for managing such cases. Understanding such concepts should promote good practice in the periodontal screening and management of orthodontic patients and enable the appropriate selection of periodontal patients suitable for orthodontic management.

Introduction

When considering the suitability of a patient for orthodontic treatment, the practitioner should consider the following questions:
• Does a malocclusion cause periodontitis?
• Can orthodontic treatment damage the periodontal tissues?
• Can orthodontic treatment be considered to manage drifting that has resulted from reduced periodontal support?

Malocclusion as a Risk Factor for Periodontitis

The concept of a "normal occlusion" does not necessarily mean a perfect Class I occlusion. Any occlusion which functions in the absence of disease, but which may also have features of malocclusion that are adequately accommodated by neuromuscular adaptation, is considered normal.

It has been estimated that 60–75% of adults in the UK have a malocclusion. Currently some 15% of orthodontic treatment is provided for adults and yet less than 15% of the population will present with severe periodontitis. Therefore a large number of adults with malocclusion appear to be free from periodontal disease. However, a proportion of adults will have both malocclusion and periodontitis and commencing orthodontic therapy in the presence of an unstable periodontium is a recipe for disaster. When the status of the periodontium is compared in teeth with and without premature occlusal contacts, no differences are found. This is evidence to suggest that malocclusion is not a primary factor in the development of a periodontal pocket.

Oral hygiene standards are a significant factor in predicting future risk of periodontitis rather than the presence of crowding and malocclusion. Where oral hygiene is good there is a minimal increase in the risk of periodontitis regardless of occlusal relationships (Fig 8-1). If oral hygiene is poor, correction of tooth alignment will not improve oral hygiene and therefore will not reduce the incidence of periodontal diseases (Fig 8-2). For patients with average oral hygiene, correction of crowding in the posterior segments may reduce the risk of periodontitis by facilitating better oral hygiene.

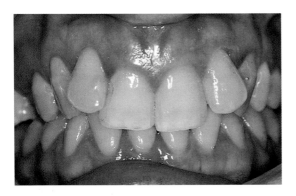

Fig 8-1 This clinical slide illustrates a patient with malocclusion. There is good oral hygiene and as a result the periodontal tissues are healthy.

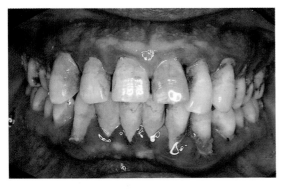

Fig 8-2 Despite a good occlusal form this patient with poor oral hygiene shows features of periodontal breakdown.

Crowded sites harbour increased quantities of supragingival plaque and raised levels of putative periodontal pathogens in subgingival locations. Correction of the malocclusion may, however, reduce levels of plaque accumulation by facilitating improved oral hygiene and reducing the risk of periodontitis by limiting the environmental risk factor of plaque accumulation. However, in a patient who is genetically susceptible to periodontitis, it is important to remember that orthodontic correction of a malocclusion will not alter their genetic susceptibility to periodontal bone loss.

The decision-making is complex, because it is essential to treat active periodontal disease and achieve stability with improved plaque control before embarking upon orthodontic therapy. Therefore, orthodontic realignment is only of benefit in cases of long-term periodontal stability in highly motivated patients. It should only be considered if patients demonstrate a stable periodontium with no progressive attachment loss for at least 9–12 months after active periodontal therapy.

Adverse Effects of Orthodontic Treatment

Orthodontic treatment may result in iatrogenic damage to teeth, temporomandibular joints and the periodontium. These potential complications rarely reach a level of clinical significance. Care in case selection, the establishment of a preventive programme and use of gentle orthodontic forces are recommended.

Caries and enamel decalcification may be found, particularly in association with fixed appliances. A daily sodium fluoride (0.05%) mouth rinse is effective in helping control caries. The dental hygienist plays a major role by providing a thorough preventive care programme, which may include topical fluoride, dietary analysis and advice, fissure sealants and oral hygiene support.

Excessive orthodontic forces may cause root resorption, which in conjunction with moderate periodontal disease can result in tooth loss at a later date (Fig 8-3).

During active orthodontic treatment, widening of the periodontal ligament space may result in increased tooth mobility. In a periodontally compromised tooth this may significantly reduce its prognosis. In general, mobility will reduce after the active stage of orthodontic therapy has been completed and the patient enters the "retention phase".

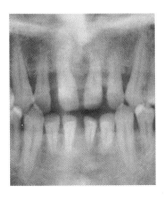

Fig 8-3 This radiograph shows severe root resorption of incisor teeth which has resulted from excessive orthodontic forces.

There is a risk of gingival recession, in particular labial to the lower incisors, when the alveolar bone plate and overlying attached gingiva are thin or where bony dehiscence or fenestrations exist. The presence of keratinised and thick overlying gingival tissue may help to prevent recession arising post orthodontic tooth movement. Gingival connective tissue grafting prior to orthodontic treatment can reduce the risk of gingival recession (Fig 8-4a, b).

A shift in the subgingival microflora occurs during orthodontic treatment. Bacteria associated with caries and periodontal diseases are found in greater numbers. Increased levels of *Streptococcus mutans,* spirochaetes, motile rods, filaments and fusiform and black pigmented *Bacteroides* sp. have been reported. Even when high standards of plaque control are maintained, orthodontic patients are likely to develop generalised gingival overgrowth and marginal gingivitis. Overgrowth is usually transient and resolves spontaneously after removal of appliances (Fig 8-5). Occasionally, fibrous hyperplasia may require surgical excision by gingivectomy or remodelling by gingivoplasty. Once again, the dental hygienist can provide invaluable support for patients during this phase of orthodontic care.

Orthodontic treatment of periodontally healthy adolescents with fixed appliances is not a major factor in influencing long-term periodontal status. Mean annual rates of attachment loss during orthodontic treatment are reported as 0.05–0.30 mm, which compares favourably with mean annual rates of attachment loss in populations not receiving orthodontic treatment.

Periodontal breakdown related to orthodontic treatment occurs in 5–10% of patients. Significantly, this mirrors the incidence of substantial periodontitis in the population as a whole. It is therefore essential to identify those

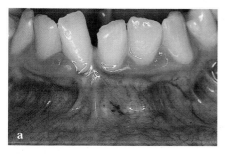 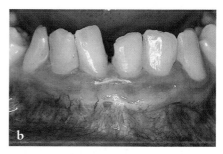

Fig 8-4(a) Patient with thin investing tissue before surgery. (b) Following connective tissue grafting to increase investing tissue during orthodontic therapy and reduce the risk of recession post orthodontics.

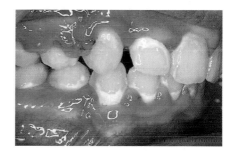

Fig 8-5 A patient undergoing orthodontic therapy with poor oral hygiene has developed gingival overgrowth.

adolescents with a high risk of periodontal disease prior to commencing orthodontic treatment. In patients for whom extractions are part of the orthodontic treatment plan, periodontal destruction is greatest at the sites of previous extractions and particularly on the pressure side of retracted canines.

Orthodontic treatment in a patient with active periodontal disease will exacerbate the rate of periodontal disease progression and significantly increase the risk of tooth loss. Conversely, a reduced but healthy periodontium, such as remains after the successful treatment of periodontitis, can be treated orthodontically without adverse effects. It is essential to make arrangements for effective periodontal maintenance (supportive care) during active orthodontic treatment of previously stabilised periodontitis patients. The dental hygienist can contribute in a significant manner to this treatment.

Orthodontic Treatment of the Periodontal Patient

Periodontal disease must be controlled prior to active orthodontic treatment and the patient should have demonstrated stability over several months of periodontal maintenance. It is essential to perform a BPE as an integral component of an orthodontic assessment.

Orthodontic treatment, in particular involving fixed appliance therapy, will contribute to increased plaque retention. In periodontal patients, a strict supportive regime for periodontal maintenance should be devised as part of the orthodontic treatment planning (Fig 8-6). This will inevitably mean more frequent visits, ideally to a dental hygienist, to check plaque control and remove soft and hard deposits during orthodontic therapy.

Consideration should be given to the extraction of teeth excluded from the arch with poor bone support, to permit alignment of the remaining dental units, e.g. lingually excluded lower incisor teeth. Loss of attachment in a reduced but healthy periodontal ligament results in a greater effect for a given orthodontic force. The orthodontist must therefore use reduced forces to limit potential damage to the periodontal ligament, cementum, alveolar bone and root dentine by resorption.

Following periodontal treatment, orthodontic treatment planning may need to be adapted to take account of the remaining, reduced periodontal tissue support. As a result of loss of alveolar bone and a reduced area of supported root structure the centre of resistance shifts apically (Fig 8-7). Teeth in such

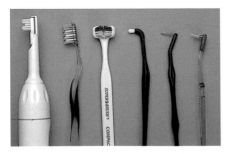

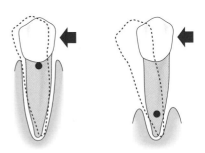

Fig 8-6 Examples of modified brushes suitable for patients with fixed appliances.

Fig 8-7 Diagram to illustrate the movement of the centre of resistance in an apical direction as periodontal bone loss occurs, rendering teeth more prone to drifting.

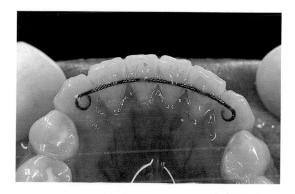

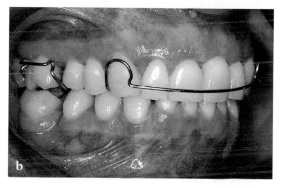

Fig 8-8(a) Clinical slide of a twist flex wire and composite splint. (b) Upper arch removable retainer designed for night time to maintain the anterior tooth alignment post-orthodontics. (c) Maryland fixed retainer placed following orthodontic treatment in a periodontal patient.

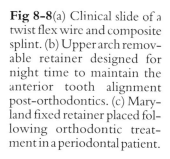

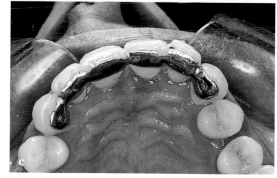

circumstances are prone to tipping, hence bodily movement requires increased reciprocating forces and moment. Permanent retention is normally required to prevent relapse (Fig 8-8a to c).

117

Key Points

- Untreated malocclusion does not contribute to an increased risk of periodontal disease, unless the patient is susceptible to periodontal disease.
- In a small number of disease susceptible patients orthodontic intervention will cause irreversible periodontal damage.
- All patients should have a BPE prior to commencing orthodontic treatment and, if necessary, detailed periodontal charting.
- Oral hygiene is the most important factor to prevent periodontal disease during orthodontic therapy.
- Adults with treated periodontal disease can safely receive orthodontic treatment, provided they have demonstrated periodontal stability during a lengthy supportive care program.
- Patients with treated periodontal disease will require intensive supportive periodontal care throughout orthodontic management.
- Oral hygiene aids specific for fixed appliance therapy will need to be introduced into the cleaning regime.
- Tooth mobility should be monitored during orthodontic therapy as this may be increased by therapy.
- When contemplating orthodontic intervention in a periodontitis patient, seek a specialist opinion in advance.
- If you suspect a patient under orthodontic care is developing periodontal complications seek early referral.

Further Reading

The Screening of Patients to Detect Periodontal Diseases. National Clinical Guidelines. London: Faculty of Dental Surgery, 1997.

Zachrisson BJ. Orthodontics and Periodontics. In: Lindhe J, Karring T, Lang NP (Eds). Clinical Periodontology and Implant Dentistry. Copenhagen: Munksgaard, 1998.

Chapter 9

Occlusion in Relation to Periodontal Disease

Aim

This chapter aims to outline the role of occlusion in periodontal disease and to identify clinical situations in which occlusal therapy may be indicated. Clinical techniques for occlusal therapy will be briefly discussed.

Outcome

Having read this chapter the practitioner should be able to recognise the influence of dynamic occlusal disharmonies on existing periodontal lesions and will have a practical understanding of how intervention may improve the prognosis of affected teeth.

Introduction

To function in occlusal harmony the masticatory apparatus comprising the teeth and supporting tissues, temporomandibular joints (TMJs) and associated neuromusculoskeletal structures must operate in an integrated and dynamic manner. Loss of integrated function or homeostasis in response to functional demand may lead to the exacerbation of an existing periodontal condition.

In health, adaptive changes occur within the periodontium to functional occlusal forces. In periodontal disease, this adaptive capacity diminishes and previously reversible changes in bone morphology may become irreversible. The ability to predict how changes may influence dental treatment is important in forecasting treatment outcomes and the longer-term prognosis for the dentition.

Normal Occlusion and the Periodontium

Teeth transmit occlusal forces generated by mastication and swallowing. The magnitude of the occlusal force is controlled by the muscles of mastication. In normal physiological function, actions last only a few tenths of a second. The direction of the majority of occlusal forces is principally axial.

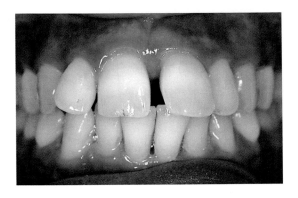

Fig 9-1 A clinical slide illustrating drifting with no periodontal disease.

The periodontium is designed to resist axial force but some lateral stress can also be tolerated.

Primary Occlusal Trauma

When persistent horizontal forces exceed the physiological limit of adaptation the periodontal fibres are unable to absorb the force and localised tissue remodelling with widening of the periodontal membrane space occurs (Fig 9-1). In the absence of periodontal disease, this is termed primary occlusal trauma. In a reduced but healthy periodontium, such as may exist after treatment of periodontal disease, forces within the normal physiological range can exceed the periodontal tissues capacity for physiological adaptation. Under such circumstances the structure and adaptive capacity of the periodontium to occlusal loading permits a degree of physiological variation in tooth mobility. The term occlusal trauma is used to describe the lesions that may develop within the periodontal tissues from occlusal disharmonies.

Clinical Features of Primary Occlusal Trauma

- No periodontitis.
- Tooth mobility in the lateral plane.
- Tooth wear (mild faceting or marked attrition) (Fig 9-2).
- Fractures of the enamel or restorations.
- Occlusal interferences (either from retruded contact position (RCP) to intercuspal position (ICP), or in lateral excursions/protrusive movements).
- Ridging of buccal mucosa.
- Indentations in lateral border of the tongue.

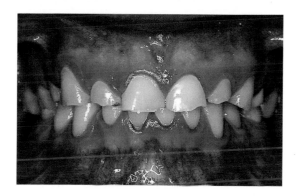

Fig 9-2 Attrition due to bruxing habit.

- Reddening of the tip of the tongue.
- Radiographically:
  - initially, widening of periodontal membrane space
  - funnel-shaped defect develops coronally in alveolus
  - hypercementosis
  - root resorption
  - secondary dentine laid down in the pulp chamber.

Management of Primary Occlusal Trauma

All pathological changes within the periodontium should be reversible and the key to successful management is to maintain periodontal health and to attempt to reduce/eliminate the excessive forces. This may involve selective grinding to remove interferences between RCP and ICP and in lateral excursion or protrusion; occlusal guards for nocturnal use (the ideal design is a "Michigan" type hard acrylic guard); and rarely splinting may be necessary to improve function (see below).

Secondary Occlusal Trauma (Trauma Within a Diseased Periodontium)

Current literature indicates that occlusal forces can cause changes in the alveolar bone and periodontal connective tissues both in the presence and in the absence of periodontitis. Secondary occlusal trauma refers to the presence of occlusal trauma in the presence of periodontitis. Secondary occlusal trauma can result in more rapid increases in tooth mobility, probing pocket depths and attachment loss. The periodontitis can be treated and periodontal health maintained without occlusal adjustment and in the presence of traumatic

121

occlusal forces. Remember, occlusal forces do not initiate periodontitis. However, in the presence of pre-existing deep periodontal pocketing, occlusal forces may in some instances act as a co-factor resulting in an increase in the rate of periodontal disease progression. The clinical features of secondary occlusal trauma are the same as for primary occlusal trauma, but additionally teeth may drift out of position and radiologically "crescentic bone loss" and angular bone defects are characteristic (Fig 9-3). In this form of occlusal trauma loading forces are within the normal physiological range. Forces acting on a reduced and inflamed periodontal attachment apparatus are therefore able to modify periodontal disease progression.

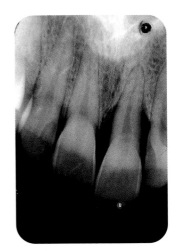

Fig 9-3 Radiograph demonstrating a crescentic pattern of bone loss 21.

Tooth mobility is a feature of occlusal overloading. However, factors other than occlusal loading contribute to the clinical observation of tooth mobility. Tooth mobility is also influenced by:
- the extent of alveolar bone loss
- the degree of attachment loss
- root length (some roots are congenitally short or pathologically shortened)
- the disruption of the periodontal tissues by inflammation.

These are essentially pathological processes whereas widening of a healthy periodontal ligament in response to occlusal forces is a physiological adaptation (Fig 9-4).

Malocclusions can potentially cause damage to:
- temporomandibular joints
- teeth by attrition (Fig 9-2)
- teeth by inducing pulpitis
- periodontal tissues by exceeding the threshold for physiological adaptation.

Occlusal features which are relevant to the risk of periodontitis
There are some specific features of malocclusion which create an increased risk of periodontal disease. When identified they should lead the practitioner to consider obtaining an orthodontic or indeed a periodontal specialist opinion.

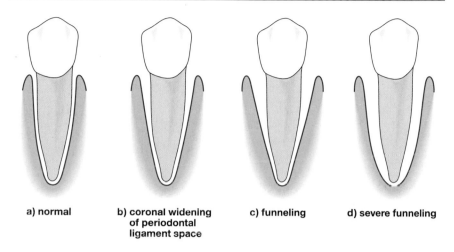

a) normal   b) coronal widening   c) funneling   d) severe funneling
of periodontal
ligament space

Fig 9-4 The sequence of change in a healthy periodontium in response to increasing occlusal loading.

Teeth which are crowded, such that they are excluded from the dental arch, are prone to localised gingival recession. Where a bone defect or dehiscence occurs and the investing tissue is thin, recession is most likely to occur. In patients with excellent manual dexterity and good oral hygiene, the control of plaque around malaligned teeth is not compromised. However, in the average patient with less than perfect oral hygiene, particularly in posterior sextants, malalignment is associated with plaque accumulation and poor periodontal status.

A deep and complete anterior overbite is a particularly destructive occlusal feature. It may cause severe shearing of the gingival tissues and food impaction labial to the mandibular incisors and palatal to the maxillary incisors. The deep anterior overbite is a feature of a Class II division 2 malocclusion. In addition, the loss of mandibular first molars can contribute indirectly to the production of a traumatic incisor relationship. Premolar and canine teeth drift distally and, in the presence of strong lower lip muscles, lower anterior teeth may retrocline into a traumatic lingual position. The lower incisors may strip the gingival tissue palatal to the upper incisors (easy to treat), or the upper incisors may strip the tissue labial to the lower incisors (difficult to treat), or both. In Class II division 1 malocclusions, only the palatal tissue is affected.

Treatment for Palatal Damage

Take study models and orthodontic advice to assess the likelihood of further eruption of the lower incisors. Reduce palatal gingival inflammation by scaling and oral hygiene instruction, and, if necessary, a gingivectomy. This may be all that is required (study models will help to see amount of tissue shrinkage). If further eruption of lower incisors is expected, make a palatal mucosal guard in metal, 3-|-3 with clasping on the canines and first premolars and reduce the lower incisors by the thickness of the guard. The guard is worn every night and one should never reduce incisors without guard construction, or they will overerupt.

Treatment for Lower Labial Damage

Scaling, root surface debridement and good oral hygiene may shrink lower labial tissue sufficiently for no further treatment to be required. Another option may be to construct an upper "Dahl" appliance (see Gough and Setchell 1999) with a solid nickel chrome platform (palatal incisal biteplane) to eliminate contact between all posterior teeth. This is believed to function by intrusion of lower incisors and an element of overeruption of posterior teeth, thereby separating the upper incisors and the lower labial gingivae. Once separation is achieved, a full upper occlusal coverage guard can be constructed from thin metal with incisal edge coverage for nocturnal use. This prevents overeruption of the upper incisors. Such cases are difficult to treat and should be referred for specialist advice/treatment. Never construct a posterior-only bite plane, as this will allow the upper incisors to overerupt and make matters worse. For severe cases, consider a combined orthodontic surgical approach.

Other Occlusal Issues

Other occlusal anomalies that may compromise periodontal health include:
- A marked increase in overjet, which is associated with increased risk of periodontal breakdown in the upper anterior sextant. However, smaller degrees of overjet not exceeding 6 mm tend to be irrelevant.
- Irregularity in the arch form will make tooth cleansing more difficult hence increasing the risk of periodontal breakdown.
- Severely rotated teeth are prone to non-axial loading forces and are frequently positioned either buccal or lingual to the arch form.
- Thin labial bone when present will predispose to local gingival recession.
- Missing and drifted teeth will also result in food trapping and plaque retention.

As periodontal breakdown occurs, occlusal interference, if present, may exceed the adaptive capacity of the residual periodontal tissues. Subsequently, tooth migration can further derange occlusal harmony. Premature molar contacts can cause forward posturing of the mandible and result in altered incisal guidance. Non-working side contacts in lateral excursion, while not causing periodontal disease, will exacerbate pre-existing periodontal defects. Such contacts are most frequently seen in the maxillary premolars. The incidence of periodontal defects is not increased in teeth with premature occlusal contact.

Following control of the active periodontal disease, occlusal therapy may be indicated if teeth remain unacceptably mobile or if the degree of mobility continues to increase.

Occlusal Therapy

Prior to embarking upon occlusal therapy, a thorough analysis must be performed. Occlusal analysis includes clinical assessment of occlusion and examination of articulated study casts. Clinical occlusal analysis should consist of a comprehensive assessment of the teeth and interarch relationships, the jaws and associated muscles, temporomandibular joints and their movements. The accurate articulation of study models is an essential component of occlusal therapy. A semi-adjustable articulator with models mounted in the retruded contact position should be employed. Examination of articulated study models allows assessment of the features of the teeth, their inter- and intra-arch arrangement, lateral guidance, faceting and patterns of tooth surface loss (see Quintessentials book *Occlusion: A Theoretical and Team Approach*).

The operator should record specific signs of occlusal dysfunction such as abrasion, attrition, localised faceting on cuspal inclines, labial drifting and overeruption of anterior teeth and increased tooth mobility. In particular, note should be made of damage to soft tissues, e.g. the palatal mucosa and lower labial gingiva. At the same time, the periodontal status should be recorded by noting sites of localised periodontal pocketing and gingival recession.

Inappropriate occlusal modification can cause irrevocable damage to the dentition. As a consequence, occlusal modifications should be practised on models before proceeding in the mouth.

Splinting in Periodontal Treatment

Splinting has very few applications in periodontally compromised dentitions. It is normally used only temporarily to stabilise teeth that require extraction in the longer term. The reason for this is that immobilisation of a tooth or removal of independent movement can result in alveolar atrophy (disuse atrophy), which for a tooth with 5–10% residual bone support can result in apical involvement. There are a few exceptions to this rule.

Splinting has limited application when inflammatory periodontal disease has been controlled. Plaque retention is a significant problem around splinted teeth and this form of management can only be used in highly motivated patients. Splinting should not be used in patients with poor oral hygiene (Fig 9-5). Splinting can be applied, if residual mobility of teeth is such that the patient finds them uncomfortable and normal masticatory function is impaired or when missing teeth require replacement and remaining teeth are unsuitable as denture or bridge abutments.

Tooth mobility is recorded using a simple index called Miller's Index:
0 = normal physiological mobility (<0.2 mm).
1 = detectable increased mobility (<1.0 mm).
2 = moderate mobility exceeding 1.0 mm.
3 = severe mobility exceeding 1.0 mm in a horizontal plane with additional vertical mobility.

Where splinting is indicated, fixed minimal preparation resin-bonded splints, e.g. twist-flex wire and composite or cast metal etch-retained structures are, the treatment of choice in periodontal patients. Splint designs incorporating some degree of individual tooth movement such as the twist-flex wire/composite system are more successful (Fig 9-6). This system has the advantage that the interdental stresses are borne by the orthodontic wire rather than directly by composite resin, which, if used alone, is likely to fracture. One solution for overcoming the interdental fracture of composite-only splints is to use glass-fibre reinforced composite (Fig 9-7). In these systems, glass fibres such as "E-glass fibres" (StickTech, Turku, Finland) can be cured within the composite to add strength to the interdental bridge, whilst still allowing some flexion and individual tooth movement. The most mobile tooth attached to a rigid splint structure is the tooth most likely to debond.

In the case of a Class II division 2 malocclusion, direct occlusal trauma may

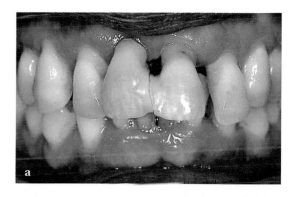

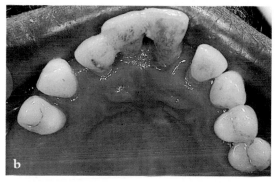

Fig 9-5 (a, b) Plaque retention with calculus around a splint.

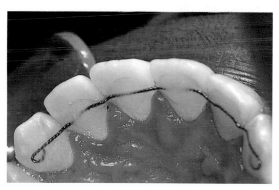

Fig 9-6 Permanent splinting using an orthodontic twist wire and palatal spot composite retention.

strip the mandibular buccal and maxillary palatal periodontal tissues from incisor teeth (Fig 9-8). A splint may offer protection for soft tissues. This is a simple alternative to complex orthodontic and orthognathic surgical management.

127

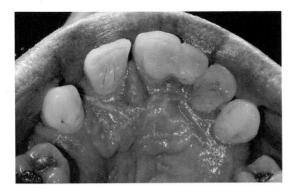

Fig 9-7 An "E-glass fibre" restoration to reduce composite fracture in the interdental zone between 21 and 22.

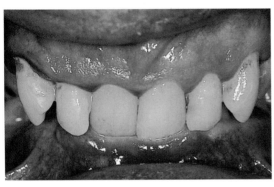

Fig 9-8 A Class II division 2 malocclusion with trauma to lower incisor periodontal support.

Following orthodontic realignment of teeth which have drifted due to periodontal disease, relapse is a significant risk. Permanent fixed splint retention is likely to be required (Fig 9-9 a, b).

Key Points

- In patients with occlusal disharmonies, occlusal therapy alone will not arrest the progression of periodontitis – periodontal therapy must take precedence over occlusal therapy.
- The decision to include occlusal adjustment as a part of periodontal therapy should follow evaluation of the patient's comfort and function.
- Occlusal therapy may have a role in the management of significant tooth mobility remaining after the control of periodontal disease, but otherwise has a minimal role in the management of periodontal patients.
- Consider referral for a specialist periodontal opinion before embarking on occlusal therapy in patients with a diagnosis of periodontitis. Mistakes

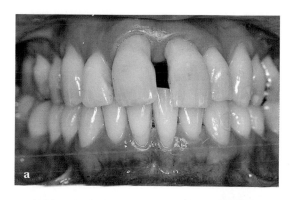

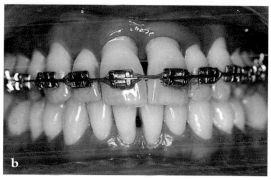

Fig 9-9 (a) Periodontal disease has been controlled but tooth drifting is a problem. (b) The same case after orthodontic alignment, permanent retention is required.

made in planning occlusal therapy in such cases can be very damaging and can alter the occlusion in an irreversible manner.

- Splinting of teeth is rarely of long-term benefit in periodontal management.

Further Reading

Gough MB, Setchell DJ. A retrospective study of 50 treatments using an appliance to produce localised occlusal space by relative axial tooth movement. Br Dent J 1999;187:134–139.

Heasman PA, Millett DT, Chapple IL. The Periodontium and Orthodontics in Health and Disease. Oxford: Oxford University Press, 1996.

Zachrisson BJ. Orthodontics and Periodontics. In: Clinical Periodontology and Implant Dentistry. Lindhe J, Karring T, Lang NP (Eds). Copenhagen: Munksgaard, 1998.

Chapter 10
Periodontal–Restorative Interface

Aim

This final chapter aims to examine the relationship between periodontal health and aspects of operative dentistry and endodontic and prosthodontic (fixed or removable) therapy.

Outcome

Having read this chapter the practitioner will appreciate why the highest standards of restorative treatment require a healthy and well-maintained periodontium with minimal gingival inflammation to facilitate good plaque control around dental restorations and appliances and thereby enhance longer-term success.

Introduction

The oral cavity is an open growth system in which most bacteria can only survive if they adhere to "non-shedding" dental hard surfaces such as teeth, restorations, dental implants or prostheses (see Chapple and Gilbert 2002). Bacterial adhesion occurs in four phases: transport to the surface, initial adhesion (which has a reversible and an irreversible stage), attachment by specific interactions and eventual colonisation. During the process of bacterial adhesion, the roughness and the free energy of the surfaces play a significant role in determining whether bacteria adhere successfully or not. A reduction in surface roughness reduces both plaque formation and maturation. A reduction in free surface energy of the substratum will result in a decrease in the plaque growth rate, a decrease in plaque retention capacity of the surface and changes in the bacterial species colonising the surface.

Intracoronal Restorations

Choice of material
The presence of any restoration in the mouth, even if of ideal quality, will increase the risk of plaque retention and, as a consequence, periodontal disease. This is for two reasons: no restorative material has a surface energy as

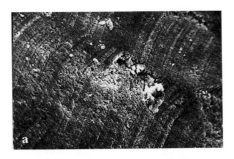
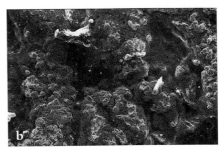
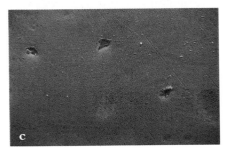

Fig 10-1 Scanning electron microscope views of (a) composite (b) amalgam and (c) gold showing different surface characteristics.

low as natural enamel and junctions between the tooth and restoration will retain plaque.

Surface roughness is an intrinsic feature of dental materials, which can be altered by polishing, scaling, brushing, condensing, glazing and finishing. A threshold surface roughness of 0.2 microns exists above which bacterial adhesion will increase. It is essential to follow manufacturer's directions for the handling and finishing of dental materials.

Whilst for anterior restorations composite materials are an aesthetic necessity, care is required in the selection of materials for posterior restorations. The surface texture of materials contributes to plaque retention (Fig 10-1 a to c). Polished gold or glazed porcelain result in minimum plaque retention, but with function even highly polished surfaces undergo wear and become more plaque retentive.

Amalgam is weakened by polishing and access to interproximal sites is difficult to achieve. The contouring of restorations and removal of marginal overhangs using diamond tips within reciprocating handpieces and conventional finishing burs are sufficient to permit adequate tooth cleaning and

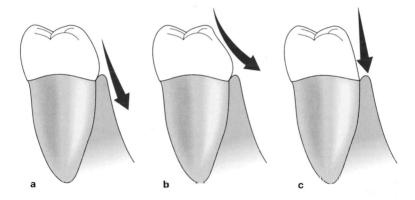

Fig 10-2 A flat emergence profile as shown in (a) mirrors natural tooth form and protects from plaque trapping that occurs in over contoured restorations (b) or physical trauma as in (c).

reduce interproximal plaque levels (see Chapple and Gilbert 2002). Polishing of amalgam restorations using rubber discs, rubber tips and polishing pastes does not result in further improvement in gingival health.

Composites can initially be finished to a suitable smooth surface texture. However, this soon deteriorates such that after six months the surface contour equates to an unfinished restoration. Plaque and gingival indices increase on older composite restorations as surface roughness and marginal seal deteriorate.

Contour
It is essential to avoid overcontouring. Bulbous restorations with wide contact areas render interproximal cleaning impossible. The concept of a flat "emergence profile" (Fig 10-2) mimicking the natural tooth contour should be followed. The use of matrix bands and wedges (Fig 10-3) will reduce the incidence of overhanging restorations (Fig 10-4). Always check that access is provided for interproximal cleaning aids. Overcontouring with direct composite additions to, for example, close spacing has been shown to increase plaque and gingival indices and probing pocket depth.

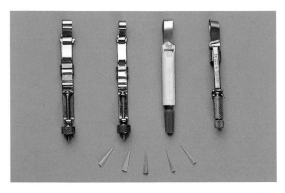

Fig 10-3 Various matrix bands and wedges used to prevent ledges on plastic restorations.

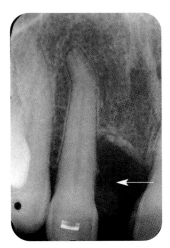

Fig 10-4 The mesial margin of 12 has been overbuilt with composite and as a result bone loss has occurred.

Marginal seal

Composite restorations are prone to marginal gap formation due to polymerisation shrinkage. This can be reduced by the incremental placement of restorations. Use of mechanical packers can improve marginal adaptation in restorations of dental amalgam.

Whenever feasible, restorations should terminate above the free margin of the gingiva. Every restoration terminating in the immediate vicinity of, or in contact with, surrounding soft tissue is a potential irritant to that tissue and increases the chance of precipitating periodontal disease. Patients with subgingival restorations will require regular dental hygiene maintenance programmes. Recurrent caries is also related to poor periodontal status (Fig 10-5).

Crowns and veneers

Material

Acrylic crowns retain plaque to a greater degree than cast gold and metal ceramic crowns. Ceramic crowns show the least plaque retention.

Margins

Crown and veneer margins are best placed in a supragingival location. Where crown height is reduced, consider crown-lengthening surgery to increase

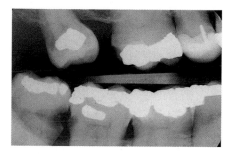

Fig 10-5 The radiograph shows recurrent caries 47, 46 and associated interproximal bone loss.

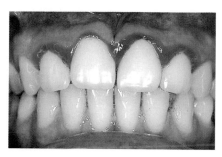

Fig 10-6 Crown margins are subgingival and inaccessible for plaque control. Gingivitis is present.

retention rather than placing margins in a subgingival location (Fig 10-6). Should crown margins be placed subgingivally, plaque retention will occur with risk of further recession. Subsequent exposure of crown margins gives a poor aesthetic outcome. If crown margins are subgingival, plaque retention and gingivitis will cause apical migration of the junctional epithelium and subsequent loss of coronal periodontal ligament fibres.

Gargiulo and colleagues proposed the existence of an innate "biological width", i.e. a minimum distance between the base of the sulcus and the most coronal periodontal fibres and alveolar bone. Based on studies of 30 cadavers, this was 2.04 mm (JE 0.97 mm, connective tissue 1.07 mm) and represents the sum of the epithelial and connective tissue

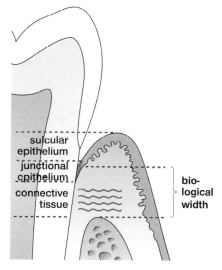

Fig 10-7 The traditional concept of the biological width is the connective tissue and epithelial attachment. Block recommends that measures be taken from the gingival margin and the biological distance be set at 3 mm (gingival margin to alveolar crest).

attachments (Fig 10-7). It is generally accepted that restorations whose margins are placed within this biological width will lead to gingival inflammation and connective tissue and bone loss. The closer a restoration margin is

135

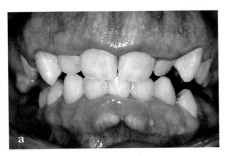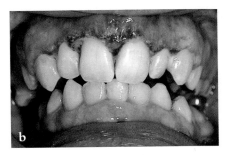

Fig 10-8 (a) Short clinical crowns. (b) 1 week following crown lengthening surgery (tissues still healing).

to the JE the more likely gingival inflammation is. The biological width described by Gargiulo et al. did not include the gingival sulcus and therefore two further recommendations have been made to help guide the clinician where to place the restoration margin:

- Ingber et al. recommended a minimal distance of 3 mm from the restoration margin to the alveolar crest, to accomodate the biological width.
- Nevins and Skurow advised that the restoration margin should not be further than 0.5–1 mm below the gingival margin.

Block, who also recommended that measures be made from the gingival margin rather than the base of the sulcus/JE because clinicians could not visualise this area, also supported the 3 mm distance. Where the margin encroached upon this distance, crown-lengthening surgery was indicated (Fig 10-8 a and b). The margins of cast ceramic restorations can be damaged during removal of investment materials and finishing. Resultant increased marginal discrepancies and eventual dissolution of cement can lead to increased plaque retention, caries and increased periodontitis.

Contour

When planning preparations for crowns and bridges, always allow adequate space for the dental technician to produce a flat emergence profile, wide interdental spaces and point contacts interproximally (Fig 10-9). These features will reduce plaque retention and allow the patient access for plaque control. This can be best achieved by laboratory techniques that conserve the gingival margin around trimmed dyes. The dental technician can then shape restorations to mimic the contour of natural teeth, which are flat at the point of contact with gingival tissue. In doing so, the overcontouring of crowns veneers and bridges is avoided (Fig 10-10).

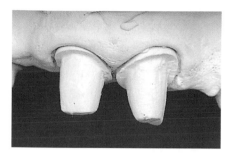 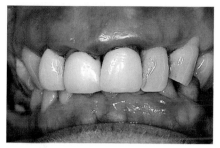

Fig 10-9 Preparation should provide the dental technician with a clear margin and tissue removal permits ideal crown contour.

Fig 10-10 A bulbous crown form that will prevent adequate plaque control.

Bridges

There is evidence that conventional bridge retainers have a significantly poor periodontal status in relation to other teeth, and that this is directly attributed to increased plaque retention. Teeth which are already compromised periodontally are not ideal as abutments for bridges.

If ideal features for crown and bridge contours are not achieved (Fig 10-11), there will be increased plaque retention with areas of potential periodontal breakdown. The ideal features include:
1. supragingival crown margins with precise marginal adaptation
2. open interdental spaces
3. point or line-shaped contact between pontic and tissue
4. ideal occlusal loading.

The profile of bridge pontics can significantly affect access for plaque control. Four pontic designs are shown in Fig 10-12. The "wash-through" design, whilst being most easily cleansable, offers poor aesthetics. The "ridge lap" design, if well polished, can be maintained plaque free with the use of superfloss.

Adhesive minimum preparation bridges
These types of restoration can be useful in the replacement of single units. In patients with periodontal disease their use can delay the need to provide a partial denture. If this can be achieved for even 5–10 years, the patient will benefit because increased risk of periodontal progression subsequent to plaque collection around partial dentures will be delayed.
There is evidence that adhesive bridges do contribute to plaque retention.

137

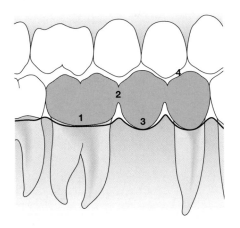

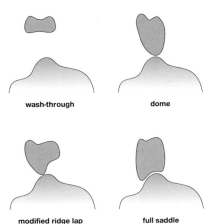

wash-through   dome

modified ridge lap   full saddle

Fig 10-11 Potential periodontal problem sites with fixed bridges (1) supragingival marginal adaptation, (2) open interdental spaces, (3) crown contour, (4) contact of pontic with tissue. Occlusal disharmony may exacerbate existing pocketing.

Fig 10-12 Diagram showing various bridge pontic designs.

Bridge abutments show statistically poorer plaque, gingivitis, recession and connective tissue attachment levels than unrestored teeth. These changes are, however, of a magnitude such that the bridges function clinically, and periodontal effects are no worse than with other forms of dental restoration. All features relating to crown construction apply to bridge design (Fig 10-13 a to d). Care is required in planning all-ceramic bridges, as connectors must be wider to permit adequate strength. It is essential to check that access is allowed for use of interproximal aids during the design of the restoration.

Implant Reconstruction

Once successful osseointegration has been achieved, implants may fail in the long term (Fig 10-14 a to d) due to overload or bacterial infection. This has been termed *peri-implantitis*. Plaque retention predisposes to peri-implantitis. Several design features of currently used implants present plaque-retentive properties. Plaque accumulation occurs:
- along the implant-transmucosal abutment interface
- at transmucosal abutment-prosthesis interfaces
- at implant-prosthesis interfaces
- on the surfaces of the implant, abutment and prosthesis.

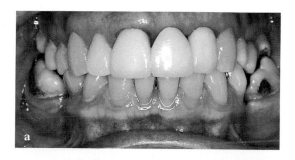

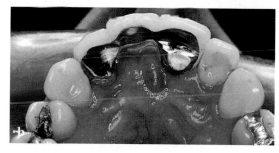

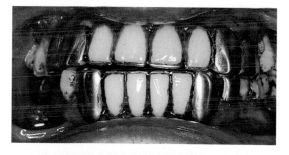

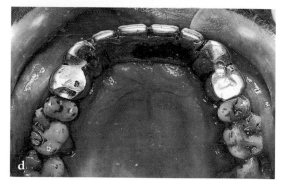

Fig 10-13 (a, b) A well-designed bridge has access for plaque control. (c, d) A poorly fabricated bridge predisposes to plaque retention.

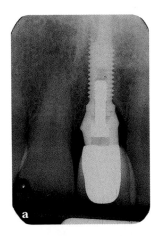

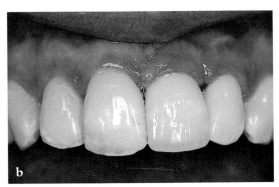

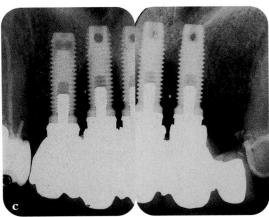

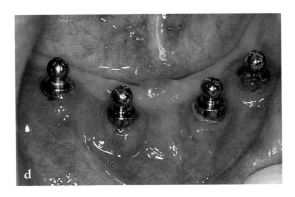

Fig 10-14 (a, b) Radiograph and clinical slide of successful implant. (c) Radiograph of failing implants in maxilla. (d) Clinical slide of failing mandibular implants.

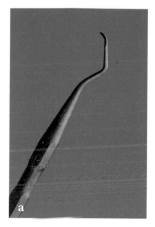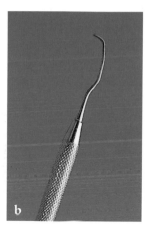

Fig 10-15 Examples of (a) plastic- and (b) gold-tipped scaling instruments for use on osseointegrated implants.

Other factors contributing to plaque accumulation are:
- size of the micro gap between the implant components
- the degree of surface roughness of restorations and abutments
- the exposure of plasma-sprayed coatings and threaded surfaces of implants
- overcontouring of implant restorations.

Care should be exercised in the use of periodontal probes around osseointegrated implants. It is possible to introduce exogenous bacteria and metal probes can scratch the implant surface thus contributing to increased plaque retention. The pocket depth surrounding an implant is not considered a valuable diagnostic criterion for the evaluation of the peri-implant condition. Probing may be difficult if the threads of screw-type implants are exposed. Patients with osseointegrated implants require a supportive care regime designed to:
- maintain periodontal health
- maintain osseointegration
- prevent the initiation or progression of soft and hard tissue lesions
- diagnose biological failures
- diagnose technical failures
- provide active therapy if indicated.

There is the potential for damage to implant surfaces when undertaking peri-implant maintenance. Ultrasonic, sonic, airbrasive, hand held stainless steel and tungsten carbide instruments can damage implants leaving roughened plaque-retentive surfaces. Implants with hydroxyapatite coatings are most susceptible to damage. Plastic- or gold-tipped instruments should be used as part of the maintenance regime (Fig 10-15 a and b).

Removable Prostheses

The breakdown of periodontal tissues in relation to removable partial dentures can be attributed to increased plaque retention and oral hygiene problems; coverage of marginal gingiva by denture components and transmission of occlusal forces by the prosthesis.

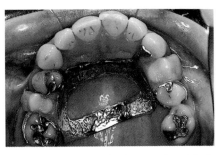

Fig 10-16 Well-designed cobalt chromium skeletally supported partial denture.

Patient compliance with oral hygiene is of greater relevance than denture design in predicting the long-term prognosis for abutment teeth affected by periodontitis. Following the removal of calculus from an acrylic denture, roughness and irregularity arise. The denture should therefore be repolished to prevent increased plaque retention. When cleaning acrylic dentures the least abrasion occurs using the lateral edge of an ultrasonic scaler tip followed by rotating silicone points in a straight hand piece.

A well-designed partial denture (Fig 10-16) has support provided by rest seats on natural teeth, positive retention provided by clasps engaging undercuts and connectors which are clear of gingival margins. A well-fitting cobalt-chromium-based denture with balanced tooth and tissue support is the ideal long-term partial prosthesis. Where remaining teeth are of doubtful prognosis or have such poor-quality residual periodontal support, such that they cannot be used to provide denture support, an acrylic mucosal supported partial denture may be considered (Fig 10-17 a and b). In designing the latter, every effort must be made to relieve the gingival margins to avoid unnecessary plaque retention or physical trauma to the gingival margins. The advantage of all-acrylic dentures is that the design allows for the addition of further teeth should they succumb to periodontal disease in the future.

Periodontal-endodontic Lesions

The periodontal tissues and the pulp-dentine complex form an intimate biological continuum through which pathological changes in either tissue may result in infection of the other. Rather than attempt to establish the primary origin of such infection, management should follow careful assessment of the viability of either or both the pulpal and periodontal tissues. Success with

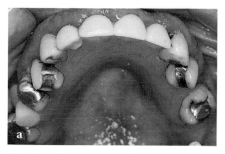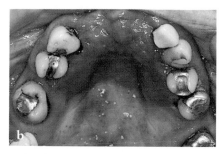

Fig 10-17 (a) An acrylic denture lacking occlusal support. (b) Denture stomatitis and poor periodontal status beneath partial denture.

therapy will only be achieved if the practitioner establishes an accurate diagnosis and follows a methodical approach to treatment planning.

The pathways of communication such as apical foramina, lateral canals, dentine tubules, root fractures, congenital grooves, root resorption and iatrogenic perforation provide a close relationship between the pulp and the periodontium. There are circumstances when endodontic treatment may cause damage to periodontal tissues. These include root canal perforation, strip perforation, post perforation and root fracture.

In general, pulpal infection has the potential to initiate inflammatory changes in the alveolus at both apical and non-apical regions of the teeth. Periodontal-endodontic lesions arise when an endodontically induced periapical lesion exists on a tooth which also has a communicating periodontal lesion (Fig 10-18). These lesions may present with either pulpal or periodontal symptoms.

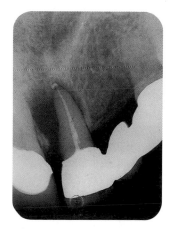

In theory, periodontal disease may lead to infection of the pulp. However, this is rare unless the periodontal lesion extends to the apical foramen. The channels for potential spread of infection from the periodontium to the pulp include lateral root canals, dentine tubules, furcation canals and resorption lacunae in areas of external resorption.

Fig 10-18 A combined periodontal endodontic lesion.

143

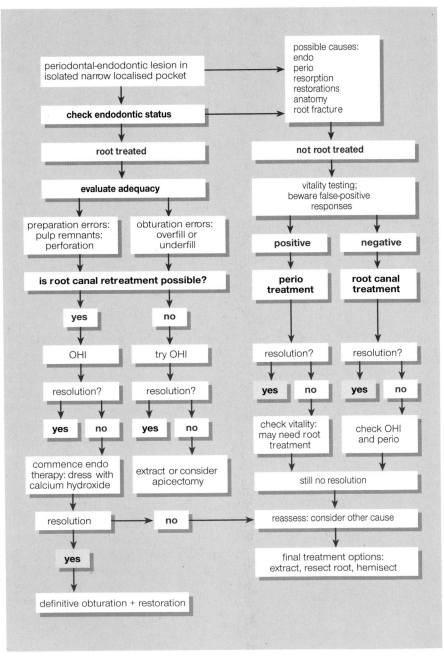

Fig 10-19 Management of combined periodontal–endodontic lesions.

A diagnosis is obtained by periodontal pocket probing, pulp vitality testing and use of periapical radiographs utilising a paralleling technique, with or without a gutta percha point placed down the sinus tract to help locate the source of infection.

The flow diagram in Fig 10-19 outlines the management of periodontal-endodontic lesions. Essentially the endodontic focus of infection must be successfully managed if such lesions are to resolve with subsequent periodontal therapies.

Management of Furcation Lesions

The presence of furcation-involved teeth in a periodontal patient will influence the treatment plan. The classification of furcation defects (Fig 10-20) is based upon the degree of periodontal destruction as assessed by pocket probing and radiographs. Furcation lesions can be classified as:

Degree I – horizontal loss of periodontal support not exceeding one-third of the width of the tooth.

Degree II – horizontal loss of periodontal support exceeding one-third of the width of the tooth, but not exceeding the total width of the furcation area.

Degree III – horizontal "through and through" destruction of the tissues in the furcation area.

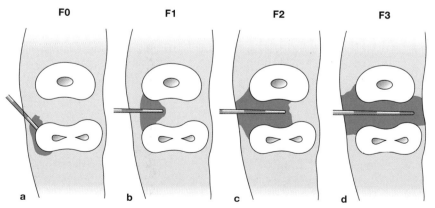

Fig 10-20 Classification of furcation defects.

Table 10-1 **Treatment options dependent upon degree of furcation involvement.**

Furcation degree	Treatment options
I	*Oral hygiene instructions Scaling and root surface debridement Furcation plasty
II	*Oral hygiene instructions Scaling and root surface debridement Furcation plasty Tunnel preparation Root resection Tooth extraction Guided tissue regeneration
III	*Oral hygiene instructions Scaling and root surface debridement Tunnel preparation Root resection Tooth extraction

* Always commence with conservative treatment, then progress if this fails.

Treatment options dependent upon the degree of furcation involvement are summarised in Table 10-1. It is essential to attempt simple therapy in the first instance.

The presence of a furcation defect adversely affects the long-term prognosis for involved teeth. Whilst simple mechanical therapy rarely results in resolution of furcation defects, it may induce recession and that may be sufficient to enable the patient to maintain the area.

Furcation plasty is a surgical technique that involves removal of root dentine at the entrance to the furcation, to open up the furcation and facilitate oral hygiene. Recession is induced and easier access for plaque control achieved.

Root resection can be performed after root canal therapy (Fig 10-21). In the maxilla, removal of the distobuccal root of molars can be considered. In the mandible, the distal root of molars normally has a circular cross-section and is the most desirable unit to retain. Alternatively, the mandibular molar roots can be sectioned and both retained as separate "premolar" units.

146

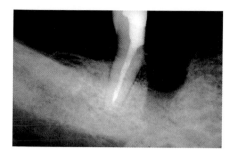

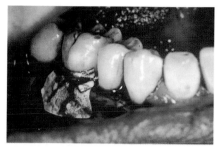

Fig 10-21 A hemi-sected tooth.

Fig 10-22 A GTR membrane at surgical placement.

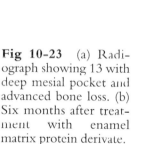

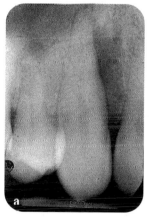

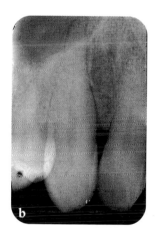

Fig 10-23 (a) Radiograph showing 13 with deep mesial pocket and advanced bone loss. (b) Six months after treatment with enamel matrix protein derivate.

Regeneration of periodontal tissues, i.e. bone, periodontal ligament and cementum can be achieved using two techniques. Guided tissue regeneration (GTR) (Fig 10-22) excludes epithelial tissue and gingival connective tissue from the healing surgical site by the use of a barrier membrane. This facilitates colonisation of the root surface with mesenchymal pluripotent stem cells capable of forming a new periodontal attachment apparatus. An alternative method relies upon the placement of enamel matrix protein on the root surface, initiating cementum formation and sequentially periodontal ligament and supporting alveolar bone (Fig 10-23 a and b). Bioceramic materials may also be used alone or with either of the two materials.

Tunnel preparation provides access to the furcation area. A tunnel preparation produces a through and through defect which the patient can access using interdental brushes. The high incidence of accessory root canals in the furcation site may result in loss of pulp vitality, which can be managed by conventional root canal therapy. Root caries is a long-term complication of this form of treatment.

Long-term retention of teeth with unmanageable furcation defects may compromise access to adjacent sites. In addition, re-infection of other residual pockets in the mouth may occur. Teeth with poor prognosis should therefore be extracted to preserve teeth with potential for long-term function. Indeed, in selected patients, a shortened dental arch, retaining only premolar, canine and incisor teeth may often be the treatment of choice.

Key Points

- Do not let your restorations be a "gilded sepulchre in the cemetery of decay", i.e. ensure a sound periodontal status prior to embarking upon operative procedures and prosthodontic treatment.
- Follow the manufacturer's directions for polishing and finishing of restorations.
- Design crowns and bridges with wide interdental spaces and flat emergence profiles.
- The dental technician can only produce ideal restorations on a well-designed preparation.
- Always give the patient specific oral hygiene advice regarding the use of interproximal cleaning aids when complex restorations are placed.
- Take care in the design of partial dentures to include support and wherever possible keep clear of the gingival margins.
- Include a supportive care regime in the treatment plan for patients with complex restorative reconstructions.

Further Reading

Al-Wahadni A, Linden GJ, Hussey DL. Periodontal response to cantilevered and fixed-fixed resin bonded bridges. Eur J Prosthodont Restorative Dent 1999;7:57–60.

Block PL. Restorative margins and periodontal health. A new look at an old perspective. J Prosthetic Dent 1987;57:683-689.

Chapple ILC, Gilbert AD. Understanding Periodontal Diseases: Assessment and Diagnostic Procedures in Practice. London: Quintessence, 2002.

Chapple ILC, Lumley PJ. The periodontal-endodontic interface. Dental Update 1999;26:331–341.

Gargiulo AW, Wentz FM, Orban B. Dimensions and relations of the dentogingival junction in humans. J Periodontol 1961;32:261–267.

Goldberg PV, Higginbottom FL, Wilson TG. Periodontal considerations in restorative and implant therapy. Periodontology 2000. 2001;25:100–109.

Meng HX. International Workshop for a Classification of Periodontal Diseases and Conditions: Periodontic-Endodontic Lesions. Ann Periodontol 1999;4:84–89.

Heasman PA, Millett DT, Chapple ILC. The Periodontium and Orthodontics in Health and Disease. Oxford: Oxford University Press, 1996.

Nevins M, Skurow HM. The intracrevicular restorative margin, the biological width and the maintenance of the gingival margin. Int J Periodontics Restorative Dent 1984;3:30-49.

O'Mahony A, MacNeill SR, Cobb CM. Design features that may influence bacterial plaque retention: a retrospective analysis of failed implants. Quint Int 2000;31:249–256.

Peumans M, Van Meerbeek B, Lambrechts P, Vanherle G, Quirynen M. The influence of direct composite additions for the correction of tooth form and/or position on periodontal health. A retrospective study. J Periodontol 1998;69:422–427.

Quirynen M. The clinical meaning of the surface roughness and the surface free energy of intraoral hard substrata on the microbiology of the supra- and subgingival plaque: results of in vitro and in vivo experiments. J Dent 1994;22 Suppl 1:S13–S16.

Renouard F, Rangert B. Risk Factors in Implant Dentistry. Chicago: Quintessence, 1999.

Index

Quintessentials for General Dental Practitioners Series

in 36 volumes

Editor-in-Chief: Professor Nairn H F Wilson

The Quintessentials for General Dental Practitioners Series covers basic principles and key issues in all aspects of modern dental medicine. Each book can be read as a stand-alone volume or in conjunction with other books in the series.

Publication date,
approximately

Oral Surgery and Oral Medicine, Editor: John G Meechan

Practical Dental Local Anaesthesia	available
Practical Oral Medicine	Spring 2004
Practical Conscious Sedation	Autumn 2003
Practical Surgical Dentistry	Spring 2004

Imaging, Editor: Keith Horner

Interpreting Dental Radiographs	available
Panoramic Radiology	Autumn 2003
Twenty-first Century Dental Imaging	Autumn 2004

Periodontology, Editor: Iain L C Chapple

Understanding Periodontal Diseases: Assessment and Diagnostic Procedures in Practice	available
Decision-Making for the Periodontal Team	Autumn 2003
Successful Periodontal Therapy – A Non-Surgical Approach	Autumn 2003
Periodontal Management of Children, Adolescent and Young Adults	Autumn 2003
Periodontal Medicine in Practice	Spring 2005

Implantology, Editor: Lloyd J Searson

Implants for the General Practitioner	Spring 2004
Managing Orofacial Pain in General Dental Practice	Spring 2004

Endodontics, Editor: John M Whitworth

Rational Root Canal Treatment in Practice	available
Managing Endodontic Failure in Practice	Autumn 2003
Managing Dental Trauma in Practice	Autumn 2003
Managing the Vital Pulp in Practice	Autumn 2004

Prosthodontics, Editor: P Finbarr Allen

Teeth for Life for Older Adults	available
Complete Dentures – from Planning to Problem Solving	Autumn 2003
Removable Partial Dentures – A Systematic Approach	Autumn 2003
Fixed Prosthodontics for the General Dental Practitioner	Autumn 2003
Occlusion: A Theoretical and Team Approach	Autumn 2004

Operative Dentistry, Editor: Paul A Brunton

Decision-Making in Operative Dentistry	available
Applied Dental Materials in Operative Dentistry	Spring 2003
Aesthetic Dentistry	Autumn 2003
Successful Indirect Restorations in General Practice	Spring 2004

Paediatric Dentistry/Orthodontics, Editor: Marie Therese Hosey

Child Taming: How to Cope with Children in Dental Practice	Spring 2003
Paediatric Cariology	Autumn 2003
Treatment Planning for the Developing Dentition	Autumn 2003

General Dentistry and Practice Management, Editor: Raj Rattan

The Business of Dentistry	available
Risk Management in General Dental Practice	Autumn 2003
Practice Management for the Dental Team	Autumn 2003
Application of Information Technology in General Dental Practice	Spring 2004
Quality Assurance in General Dental Practice	Autumn 2004
Evidence-Based Care in General Dental Practice	Spring 2005

Quintessence Publishing Co. Ltd., London